Clinical Documentation Improvement

Ruthann Russo, PhD, JD, MPH, RHIT

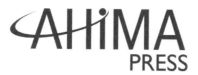

AHIMA
PRESS

ISBN 978-1-58426-226-8

AHIMA Product No. AB121608

AHIMA Staff:
Claire Blondeau, MBA, Senior Editor
Cynthia Douglas, Developmental Editor
Katie Greenock, Editorial and Production Coordinator
Ashley Sullivan, Assistant Editor
Jill S. Clark, MBA, RHIA, Reviewer
Kathryn DeVault, RHIA, CCS, Reviewer
Ken Zielske, Director of Publications

All information contained within this book, including Web sites and regulatory information, was current and valid as of the date of publication. However, Web page addresses and the information on them may change or disappear at any time and for any number of reasons. The user is encouraged to perform his or her own general Web searches to locate any site addresses listed here that are no longer valid.

AHIMA strives to recognize the value of people from every racial and ethnic background as well as all genders, age groups, and sexual orientations by building its membership and leadership resources to reflect the rich diversity of the American population. AHIMA encourages the celebration and promotion of human diversity through education, mentoring, recognition, leadership, and other programs.

American Health Information Management Association
233 North Michigan Avenue, 21st Floor
Chicago, Illinois 60601-5800

http://www.ahima.org

Brief Contents

Detailed Table of Contents

About the Author

Ruthann Russo, PhD, JD, MPH, RHIT, has worked in the health information management arena since 1980, spending time in a variety of areas including quality assurance, HIM, academics, and consulting. She has founded two successful, award-winning consulting firms and currently is a faculty member teaching complementary and integrative medicine and the director of clinical affiliations and the community connections program for tri-state college of Acupuncture in New York City. She is also managing director with Navigant Consulting's Healthcare Group.

Dr. Russo is the author of nine books and many articles, papers, and presentations on topics spanning the HIM, healthcare, and management disciplines. She has written scripts for and appeared in several video presentations on CDI, reimbursement, and HIM compliance, appeared on radio programs, and participated in several audio conferences for AHIMA and other healthcare organizations.

Dr. Russo received her BA from Dickinson College, her JD from American University, her MPH from the Robert Wood Johnson Medical School/University of Medicine & Dentistry of New Jersey, and her PhD from Touro University.

Introduction
The Importance of Clinical Documentation in Today's Healthcare Environment

Patient Care and Quality

Clinical documentation, a term that is used frequently and freely in the healthcare industry, is a term that has escaped a consistent definition to date. For purposes of this book, clinical documentation is any manual or electronic notation (or recording) made by a physician or other healthcare clinician related to a patient's medical condition or treatment. This book presents an objective and uniform set of clinical documentation principles that can be applied reliably throughout the industry.

Quality is another term commonly used in healthcare. It is also a term that has escaped precise definition. Quality clinical documentation, as explained in chapter 1, meets seven criteria:

- Legible
- Reliable
- Precise
- Complete
- Consistent
- Clear
- Timely

Clinical documentation is the foundation of every patient health record. By creating records for the patients they treat, healthcare organizations are in essence, medical trustees for their patients' protected health information. Since the dawn of the Health Information Portability and Accountability Act (HIPAA), both patients and the organizations that treat them are beginning to appreciate the critical value of that information even more. The next challenge for the healthcare industry is ensuring consistency in content and meaning of clinical information as it evolves from a manual to an electronic practice. The subsequent challenge, being tackled by a few visionary healthcare systems right now, is digitally compiling all health information about one patient into a common location. The electronic health record has the potential of creating significant positive impact on healthcare quality—but *only* if the information in the record is itself of the highest possible quality.

High-quality clinical documentation and the need for a structure to continuously support the function are the premise for this book. High-quality clinical documentation is the goal of every clinical documentation improvement (CDI) program. However, because a common definition for what constitutes high-quality clinical documentation across the healthcare industry is currently lacking, this book proposes standardized criteria. Implementation, operationalization, and continued maintenance of a healthcare organization's clinical documentation management program are described in detail in three sections of this book. Part 1 addresses the fundamentals of clinical documentation including assessing the current quality of a healthcare organization's clinical documentation and making the decision to move forward with a new program or adding improvements to the current program. Part 2 describes the clinical documentation program implementation from staffing the program through training and querying physicians, analyzing program data, and ensuring program compliance. Finally, part 3 recommends and explains a process for growing and refining a clinical documentation program. The book ends, as it begins, with a focus on the patient, specifically addressing the possibility of involving patients in the CDI process.

The Users of Health Information

The vast and myriad uses and users of health information illustrate the importance of the health records that house that information. The record benefits the patient, but, it can also benefit many other patients when that information is used for research purposes. Furthermore, the health information derived from clinical documentation in the record drives the decision-making process of the healthcare industry for providers and payers alike. In fact, the information in a patient's record is the common ground shared by everyone who is involved in or touches the healthcare industry. Patients, the government, physicians, pharmaceutical firms, insurers, research organizations, healthcare systems, and other providers all need the information in patient health records to fulfill their responsibilities. It is important to define each of these users of health information and how they benefit individually from the information as well as how they contribute to the overall larger body of health information.

Patients

Without the patient, there *is* no health record. The primary purpose for maintaining a health record is to "accurately and adequately document a patient's life and health history, including past and present illness(es) and treatment(s), with emphasis on the events affecting the patient during the current episode of care" (Huffman 1994, 30). The health record is the primary reference tool for all physicians and clinicians treating the patient. Clinical documentation, which is the foundation of the patient's record, is the key factor in determining the quality of care provided to the patient.

It is also important for patients to know that the quality of their health information depends upon their responses to questions the physician and other clinicians ask them during a visit. Patients who are prepared to answer questions about their symptoms accurately provide clinicians with better raw material to work with in their own documentation.

To patients, information in the health record can be difficult to understand. Yet, patients who learn some basic facts and become familiar with the record will be more empowered than patients who are uninformed about their health information. The knowledgeable and proactive patient is also likely to respond to questions with greater accuracy.

HIPAA has raised awareness about patients' rights concerning their health information. As a result, more patients are likely to request copies of their records. HIPAA has also increased the popularity of the electronic health record. The act of reading, understanding, and asking questions about health information creates healthcare consumers who are better decision makers and participants in their own care. And, when patients are proactive participants with healthcare planning, and they understand the importance of their health information, their providers are likely to be more accountable for the quality of information they document in the health record.

Physicians and Other Clinicians

The health record is the primary tool for clinicians to communicate with each other about a patient. As the next example shows, a patient will be treated by seven different clinicians during an average acute care hospital stay. The typical hospital record includes entries made by the attending physician, specialists, house staff (for teaching hospitals), nurses, radiologists, pathologists, and therapists. The inaccurate or unreliable clinical documentation of one provider can create a domino effect that negatively impacts the quality of care provided to the patient. While the importance of clinical documentation is clear to most physicians and they agree, when surveyed, that they should practice high-quality clinical documentation, medical school students, residents, and most clinicians are not thoroughly trained in the principles of high-quality clinical documentation. This gap necessitates that hospitals and healthcare systems fill the void by providing comprehensive and consistent training in clinical documentation as well as ongoing support through a structured clinical documentation program.

Healthcare Provider Organizations

Clinical documentation quality determines the quality of a healthcare manager's decision-making ability. As a result, health records and the clinical documentation contained in them may be the most valuable asset of a healthcare organization. Individually, these records are the basis for payment for all services provided by healthcare organizations. Each record is evidence that the care billed for was in fact provided to the patient. In aggregate, health records create a data set that healthcare organizations rely upon for strategic and financial planning, budgeting, and internal research. A hospital's senior management team can trend treatment and resource needs, staffing requirements, and disease patterns by reviewing the diagnostic data gleaned from the clinical documentation in patients' records. In addition, hospitals can purchase the data of other hospitals to run comparative analyses. The results of these analyses can help the management team determine future demand for services in their market so they can better prepare. The trustworthiness of management decisions in the healthcare industry is directly proportional to the quality of the clinical documentation in patient records.

Insurers

Insurers pay for care that was provided to their subscribers subject to the policy limitations. However, because no plan will pay for care that was not provided, most insurers perform regular audits of documentation in patient health records. If the clinical documentation in the record does not support the bill for services, the insurer will reject the bill outright. Clinical documentation in patient records is also used by insurers for precertification or preapproval of services like MRIs or surgery. Inaccurate clinical documentation in this situation can mean a denial of service, and the patient may not receive a necessary test or treatment.

Government and Regulatory Agencies

This category includes federal and state government agencies as well as organizations like The Joint Commission, HealthGrades, the LeapFrog Group, and other organizations that publish healthcare quality ratings. State and federal governments, when acting as an insurer for Medicare or Medicaid recipients, have the same interests and responses as the insurers. However, the government also plays a regulatory role in measuring and attempting to ensure a certain level of quality in healthcare. At the federal level, the Medicare quality indicators (http://www.cms.hhs.gov/QualityInitiativesGenInfo/15_MQMS.asp) play an important role in comparative measurement among healthcare organizations.

Accreditation organizations also produce measures that are used by healthcare consumers and insurers to select healthcare providers. To some degree, all quality measurements rely upon clinical documentation in patient records and the resulting coded data. Measures like Healthgrades rely entirely on data derived from clinical documentation in health records to assign quality ratings to hospital care, while CMS's quality indicators are driven by a combination of data and original clinical documentation. The bottom line is that quality measures that consumers use to make the best decisions about their healthcare are only reliable to the extent that the clinical documentation in patient records is of high quality.

Research Organizations and the Pharmaceutical Industry

A large percentage of clinical documentation research is sponsored by research organizations and the pharmaceutical industry. Researchers rely on clinical documentation in two primary ways. First, the health records of patients participating in research studies are scrutinized by the researchers. Second, the ICD-9-CM data derived from clinical documentation in patient health records is utilized by hospital- and academic-based researchers to identify successful treatment trends and changes in disease patterns. This data may also be used to support hypotheses and design new research studies. The validity of hypotheses and research studies is only as accurate as the clinical documentation in patient records.

The Need for High Quality Clinical Documentation

This overview of the users and uses of health information demonstrates the crucial need for high-quality clinical documentation in patient records. The need starts with the individual patient and then impacts most healthcare consumers as well as industries. Current gaps in the clinical documentation process that this book attempts to fill include the lack of a consistent criteria set and the lack of a standardized training system for high-quality clinical documentation. In addition, the book presents suggestions for design, implementation, and continued renewal of a clinical documentation program. It is imperative that healthcare providers and professionals standardize the way they measure the quality of clinical documentation for the benefit of patients, physicians and clinicians, and the entire healthcare industry.

References

Huffman, E.K. 1994. *Health Information Management*. Berwyn, IL: Physicians Record Company.

Part 1
Fundamentals of Clinical Documentation

Chapter 1
Criteria for High-Quality Clinical Documentation

The Need for High Quality Clinical Documentation

High-quality clinical documentation is a necessary but still uncommon practice within today's healthcare communities. It is a practice that all healthcare organizations need and want, yet few are able to achieve completely. This chapter first presents the research findings that support the proposition that high-quality clinical documentation does not exist today in most healthcare organizations. Then, a theory of high-quality clinical documentation is described, followed by an explanation of seven criteria for high-quality clinical documentation. These criteria and the proposed theory are then supported by peer-reviewed research results, as well as healthcare laws and regulatory guidelines. Ultimately, it is the sharing and reinforcing of this information with physicians and clinicians in provider organizations that turns the theory into practice and results in real impact on the quality of clinical documentation.

Evidence to Support the Lack of High-quality Clinical Documentation

The current research available on clinical documentation reveals that lack of adequate documentation is a problem throughout the healthcare industry (Cascio et al. 2005, 346; Novitsky et al. 2005, 627). The peer-reviewed academic literature also shows a relationship between documentation and quality of care, as well as support for concurrent clinical documentation improvement programs. Reasons for poor quality clinical documentation identified in the research include:

- Clinical documentation practices are not taught in medical school or residency programs.
- The importance of physician clinical documentation is not a top priority for healthcare organizations.
- The information, especially in the inpatient setting, is complex.
- Increased length of stay and multiple providers are common.
- Unstructured or inconsistent processes for recording and collection of information are prevalent.

The following is a brief synopsis of the current peer-reviewed research published on the challenges associated with attaining high-quality clinical documentation.

Over the past two decades, researchers have found quality problems in physician documentation in many parts of the health record including progress notes, history and physical reports, problem lists, and operative notes. In addition, one study found significant discrepancies between orthopedic surgeon office notes and hospital notes for the same patient. An overview of the studies by type of documentation problem follows (Russo 2007).

Deficiencies in documenting history and physical exams were studied by both the Cascio and Bachman teams. In the Cascio study, the researchers focused on clinical documentation specific to the clinical course of acute compartment syndrome. The term compartment syndrome refers to increased tissue pressure within a closed fascial space, resulting in tissue ischemia (Beers 2006).

In this study, documentation was found to be inadequate for 70 percent of the patient records. Notes and consent forms for 30 consecutive patients with adequate follow-up who had undergone fasciotomy for the treatment of compartment syndrome were reviewed for legibility, notation of the time and date, and documentation of the presence of core physical examination and history findings, including pain, paresthesias, tenseness, pain on passive stretch, sensory deficit, motor deficit, pulses, compartment pressures, and diastolic blood pressure (Cascio et al. 2005, 346). Here, the researchers found that thorough documentation can contribute to the identification of subtle changes in the physical examination findings, which may aid in increased quality of care to the patient. The researchers further note that a possible reason for the widespread lack of proper documentation is a lack of emphasis on careful documentation in medical schools, residency programs, and physician practices (Cascio et al. 2005, 346).

Bachman's research on the patient interview process and documentation of that process revealed that physicians often omit questions, diagnoses, or other important information in the documentation of the patient's history and physical examination. In Bachman, the researchers' review of the physician history-taking process revealed that the process is often incomplete as well as time consuming. Here, the researchers performed a review of literature to identify the importance of the use of a checklist in obtaining and documenting a patient's history. They also compared the use of a checklist by a physician to the use of a checklist by an airplane pilot—claiming that just as a pilot would not take off without reviewing his checklist, so a physician should not treat a patient without reviewing his checklist (Bachman 2003, 67).

The Carroll research team found documentation discrepancies in 62 percent of the progress notes reviewed. These researchers conducted a review of resident physicians' progress notes over 40 random days in a four-month period in a neonatal intensive care unit. Using predetermined criteria, they assessed the reliability of medications, vascular lines, and patient weights. Discrepancies occurred in the documentation of medications in 28 percent of progress notes, of vascular lines in 34 percent of progress notes, and of weights in 13 percent of progress notes. In this study, patients with more medications or vascular lines, and with longer lengths of stay, were significantly more likely to have higher rates of documentation errors. The study concluded that daily progress notes written by resident physicians in the neonatal intensive care unit often contained inaccurate, or omitted pertinent, information (Carroll et al. 2003, 976).

Carroll identified that clinical documentation errors are common in healthcare settings where the patient stays are longer and complicated. This finding supports giving top priority to inpatient acute care heath records when undertaking a clinical documentation program. In addition, the researchers found that when the documentation was not provided by the physician immediately after care was given, the quality of the documentation in the patient's record was susceptible to neglect and data loss (Stengal et al. 2004, 553). This finding supports the key activity of a clinical documentation program as being concurrent review and concurrent physician inquiry. In this study, physicians themselves also identified that they were not always able to access the information they were seeking in the patient's record to help treat the patient. These physicians attributed the reasons for their inability to access such information to illegible handwriting, too little time, and disorganized charts.

The quality of problem list documentation was addressed by three different research teams: Spencer, Sabinis, and Weitzel. The Spencer research demonstrated that current smoking status, an important data element in measuring patient quality of care under the Medicare quality indicators, was often not documented in the problem list within the patient's record. Although the problem list is a major document in the patient record, relatively easy to understand and complete, physicians often omitted current smoking status or did not complete the form at all (Spencer et al. 1999, 18).

In the Sabinis study, education and informational sessions were used to increase the likelihood that a physician would document the vaccination status of patients. In the case of documentation of childhood sexual abuse, it was found that tailored feedback to the physician with directed educational materials improved most aspects of documentation and knowledge of childhood sexual abuse. The Socolar study on the documentation of childhood sexual abuse found that continuing medical education and a structured record were consistently associated with better documentation. The Humphreys study showed that the use of templates can improve documentation in the emergency department (Humphreys et al. 1992, 534).

The Weitzel study revealed that 49 of 49 items were completed on mental status examinations when a checklist was used, whereas only 4 of 49 items were completed when no checklist was used. While a checklist can be an important part of documentation collection, it will not resolve the majority of clinical documentation challenges and should only be a partial strategy. In addition, there may be compliance concerns with use of checklists, so the specific format would need to be reviewed and approved by the organization's compliance and legal groups prior to use. A checklist cannot be used, for example to ensure that a physician documents the clinical significance of every abnormal test result in a patient's record (Weitzel and Waller 1990, 23–34).

The Manfield study identified that a patient's hospital health record often lacked significant amounts of clinical documentation that were frequently contained in the orthopedic surgeon's office-based record for that patient. In this case, the orthopedic surgeons appeared to be less concerned about the documentation in the hospital record than they were about the documentation in their own office health records (Manfield et al. 2001, 51).

The Devon and Novitsky research teams found problems with the quality of physician operative notes. The Devon study found that the patient's health record was an inaccurate and inadequate source of information about symptoms experienced by patients with acute myocardial infarctions. Operative notes dictated by surgeons were found to contain numerous deficiencies. In a teaching-hospital setting, operative notes dictated by attending physicians were found to contain fewer deficiencies than operative notes dictated by residents, but in both cases there was a significant failure to produce high-quality operative notes (Devon 2004, 547).

Novitsky found that residents were in error in 28 percent of the operative reports that they dictated. Accurate and complete operative reports are essential for medical and legal purposes, and they also serve as an important communication tool for all healthcare personnel involved in the care of a particular patient. These dictations delineate operative indications and justify the surgery. In addition, a full description of positive and negative findings, as well as the thought process behind them, may influence not only the quality of care for the patient, but also the outcome of a malpractice lawsuit (Novitsky et al. 2005, 627).

Evidence-based Documentation: The Theory of High-quality Clinical Documentation

Because clinical documentation in patient health records is highly regulated, any theory concerning it must begin with regulatory and legal requirements. Medicare Conditions of Participation requires all healthcare providers to maintain patient health records and dictates certain content. In addition, the Department of Health and Human Services' Office of the Inspector General (OIG) guidance recommends the following minimum compliance for health record documentation:

1. The health record should be complete and legible.

2. Past and present diagnoses should be accessible in the health record.

3. Appropriate health risk factors should be identified.

4. If not documented, the rationale for ordering diagnostic and ancillary services should be easily inferred by an independent reviewer.

5. The patient's progress and his response to any changes in treatment and any revision in diagnoses should be documented.

6. Documentation of each patient encounter should include the reason for the encounter with any relevant history, physician examination findings, prior diagnostic test results, assessments, clinical impressions, diagnoses, plan of care, date of service, and legible identity of the observer (Adams et al. 2002).

Government, regulatory, and accreditation resources for health record content are shown in figure 1.1.

The theory of high-quality clinical documentation is a two-part, cause and effect theory. The first part of the theory, which identifies criteria for high quality, is derived from legal and regulatory sources. The second part of the theory is derived from the peer-reviewed research discussed earlier in this chapter. The theory of high-quality clinical documentation states that *if* the seven criteria of high-quality clinical documentation

Figure 1.1   Resources for health record content

- Medicare Conditions of Participation
  http://www.cms.hhs.gov/CFCsAndCoPs/06_Hospitals.asp
- The Joint Commission
  http://www.jointcommission.org/
- PRO Directory
  http://www.ahqa.org/pub/connections/162_694_2450.cfm
- Official Guidelines for Coding and Reporting (CDC)
  http://www.cdc.gov/nchs/data/icd9/icdguide.pdf
- OIG—3rd Party Billing Guidance (p.7—fn.48–51)
  http://oig.hhs.gov/fraud/docs/complianceguidance/thirdparty.pdf

are applied to clinical documentation, *then* clinical documentation quality will be high and the accuracy of care, quality indicators, reimbursement, healthcare planning, and research (the activities that clinical documentation impacts) will be improved.

Evidence-based medicine (EBM) means practicing medicine using only the best scientific data available. Just as in medical practice, physicians should only be practicing clinical documentation using the best scientific data available. *A Compelling Case for Clinical Documentation,* describes in detail the interventional study, performed with controls and conducted with medicine residents, used to test the first part of the theory of high-quality clinical documentation (Russo 2008). The study found a statistically significant relationship between training in the seven criteria for high-quality clinical documentation and improvement in the quality of the physicians' clinical documentation (Russo and Fitzgerald 2008). The study was peer reviewed by the Academy of Management and nominated for a Best Theory to Practice Award. Because of the peer-reviewed research support for the theory of high-quality clinical documentation, if physicians and clinicians practice clinical documentation using these established standards, they are practicing evidence-based documentation.

In *The Gold Standard: The Challenge of Evidence-Based Medicine and Standardization of Health Care,* the authors use the evolution of patient health records as an analogy for evidence-based medicine. EBM is about creating a standard in medical care. There are four kinds of standards used in EBM: design, terminology, performance, and procedural (Timmermans and Berg 2003). The authors point out that the notion of patient-centered health record keeping, which had begun in the U.S. at the turn of the 20th century, like EBM, also encompassed all four types of standardization. Additionally, they describe the evolution of patient record-keeping standards from the 1920s, when the American College of Surgeons was the only regulating body for health record content, to today's rigorous requirements of Medicare, The Joint Commission, and state departments of health.

Criteria for High-quality Clinical Documentation

The seven criteria for high-quality clinical documentation require that all entries in the patient record be:

1. Legible
2. Reliable
3. Precise
4. Complete
5. Consistent
6. Clear
7. Timely

The first six criteria are focused on in a review process because, if necessary, they can be corrected after the fact; however, the last, timeliness, is one criterion that cannot be corrected after the fact since once an entry is late, it remains late. The following are the seven criteria for high-quality clinical documentation (Russo and Fitzgerald 2008; Russo 2007). The initial definition provided for each criterion is taken from the *Oxford English Dictionary* (6th edition, 2005). Following the dictionary definition is a description of how the criteria can be applied to patient health record documentation. Examples of documentation that do and do not meet the criteria are also included after each definition with the exception of legibility and timeliness.

Legible

Clear Enough to Be Read and Easily Deciphered

The inability to read a record entry is usually due to the fact that the physician's handwriting is indecipherable. Legibility is addressed as a requirement for clinical documentation by every regulatory body and law that addresses health record content. The most recent nod to the importance of legibility came when HIPAA gave patients the right to ask for clarification of illegible information in their records. Illegible handwriting is usually the result of a rushed or careless documentation practice. As the electronic health record (EHR) evolves, handwriting becomes less of an issue. However, there are other risks inherent in the rushed or careless use of an EHR that may cause the definition of legibility to be amended for these purposes.

Reliable

Trustworthy, Safe, Yielding the Same Result When Repeated

This criteria relates to treatment provided to the patient and whether the physician's documentation supports the treatment. For example, a physician orders a blood transfusion for a patient who has an upper gastrointestinal bleed and severely low hemoglobin and hematocrit levels. The physician's diagnosis for the patient is a bleeding gastric ulcer. The physician's diagnosis of a bleeding gastric ulcer does not appear to be reliable based on the treatment given. Blood transfusion is not an accepted treatment for a gastric ulcer. If the physician documents bleeding gastric ulcer with acute blood loss anemia (if clinically indicated), based on the treatment given, this is a reliable diagnosis.

Documentation That Does Not Meet Reliability

Patient is admitted with shortness of breath and chest pain. The patient is treated with Lasix, oxygen, and Theophylline. The physician's final documented diagnosis for the patient is acute exacerbation of chronic obstructive pulmonary disease (COPD).

Documentation That Does Meet Reliability

The patient was given Lasix to treat an acute and chronic congestive heart failure (CHF). The physician amends the final progress note to reflect the final diagnosis: Acute exacerbation of chronic bronchitis and COPD; acute and chronic CHF. In this case, the patient had bronchitis with the COPD, so the initial documentation did not meet criteria for both reliability and precision.

Precise

Accurate, Exact, Strictly Defined

Detail, if available and clinically appropriate, is an important component of every patient's health record. The more detailed the physician's documentation, the more representative and accurate the clinical documentation in the patient's record is likely to be.

Documentation That Does Not Meet Criteria for Precision

Patient is admitted with chest pain, shortness of breath, fever, and cough. Chest x-ray shows aspiration pneumonia. The physician's final documented diagnosis for the patient is pneumonia.

Documentation That Meets Criteria for Precision

The physician reviews the chest x-ray and documents the patient's final diagnosis in the discharge summary as *aspiration pneumonia*.

Complete

Having the Maximum Content, Thorough

This means that the physician has fully addressed all concerns in the patient record. Completeness also includes the appropriate authentication by the physician or clinician, which generally includes a signature and a date. Diagnostic documentation concerns apply to anything from the patient's initial complaint (did the physician provide a working and final diagnosis?) to ordering of tests (did the physician document the reason for the tests?) to abnormal diagnostic test results (did the physician document the clinical significance of any abnormal diagnostic test?)

Documentation That Does Not Meet Criteria for Completeness

Physician orders comprehensive blood chemistries. The tests show low sodium levels, low magnesium levels, and low potassium levels. The physician does not document diagnoses to represent any of these abnormal results, nor does he document that the results are clinically insignificant.

Documentation That Meets Criteria for Completeness

In the previous example, the physician documents the following in the patient's progress notes on the day after the test results were received:

> *Na 131 Mg 1.3 K+ 3.1; Patient dehydrated. Potassium within normal limits. Patient given CAD and hypertensive medication.* The physician should not document a diagnosis if the clinical evidence did not support it. However, if the abnormal test results do not support a diagnosis, then the physician should document, *"abnormal test results are clinically insignificant."*

Consistent

Not Contradictory

Clinical documentation about a patient that contradicts itself from one progress note to the next or among entries from different physicians is a documentation deficiency. The overall rule is that when another physician's documentation conflicts with the attending physician's documentation, and the attending is unavailable to state otherwise, the attending physician's documentation takes precedence. However, if the attending physician has provided documentation that appears to contradict itself, he must clarify and add an addendum to the discharge summary or a final progress note.

Documentation That Does Not Meet Criteria for Consistency

Patient is admitted by her primary care physician with vertigo and confusion. The primary care physician documents the patient's preliminary diagnosis as TIA and asks for a neurology consult. The neurologist examines the patient and documents the diagnosis in his final consultation as cerebrovascular accident (CVA). The attending physician provides no further documentation regarding the patient's diagnosis. (In this case, the attending physician and the neurologist's diagnoses are inconsistent).

Documentation That Meets Criteria for Consistency

The attending physician is asked to rereview the neurologist's consultation. The attending physician adds a final progress note to the patient's record that states the final diagnosis is *CVA*.

Clear

Unambiguous, Intelligible, Not Vague

Vagueness and ambiguity exist when the clinical documentation does not totally describe what is wrong with the patient. This may result in the documentation of symptoms without etiology or possible etiology. For example, if a patient presents with a symptom such as chest pain and the physician provides no other insight in his documentation, it would be considered vague. If there is no clinical evidence for any diagnosis, then the appropriate documentation would be, "*chest pain etiology undetermined.*"

Documentation That Does Not Meet Criteria for Clarity

Patient presents with syncope. The physician orders a CT scan and MRI of the brain, EKG, and blood tests, all of which are within normal limits. The physician's final diagnosis on discharge is syncope.

Documentation That Meets Criteria for Clarity

In the previous example, the following documentation would meet criteria for clarity, assuming that the appropriate clinical indicators were present:

1. Syncope, etiology undetermined

2. Syncope, possible bradycardia

3. Syncope, probable transient ischemic attack (TIA)

Timely

At the Right Time

Timeliness of clinical documentation is essential to the best treatment of the patient. The EHR can help with timeliness, but the clinician's input is still necessary. In addition to daily progress note entries and timely discharge summaries, physicians also need to be timely with diagnoses that are present on admission. Hospitals need to report when a diagnosis was present on admission as evidence that the condition did not develop in the hospital. Present on admission documentation impacts research, reimbursement, quality indicators, and planning.

Table 1.1 provides a summary of criteria for high-quality clinical documentation with representative examples.

Conclusion

High-quality clinical documentation is necessary for every healthcare organization. In order to achieve high-quality clinical documentation on a national level, it is necessary for healthcare providers to use a standardized set of guidelines and definitions. This chapter presents a theory of high-quality clinical documentation supported by peer-reviewed research and healthcare laws and regulations as a first step in helping providers to develop a high-quality clinical documentation practice.

Table 1.1.   Documentation criteria

Criteria for High Quality Clinical Documentation	Example/Description
Legibility	Required under all government and regulatory agencies
Completeness	Abnormal test results without documentation for clinical significance (Joint Commission requirement)
Clarity	Vague or ambiguous documentation, especially in the case of a symptom principal diagnosis (chest pain vs. GERD or syncope vs. dehydration)
Consistency	Disagreement between two or more treating physicians without obvious resolution of the conflicting documentation upon discharge
Precision	Nonspecific diagnosis documented, more specific diagnosis appears to be supported (anemia vs. acute or chronic blood loss anemia)
Reliability	Treatment provided without documentation of condition being treated (Lasix, no CHF documented; KCI administered, no hypokalemia documented)

References

Adams, D. L., H. Norman, and V.J. Bourroughs. 2002. Addressing medical coding and billing part two: A strategy for achieving compliance. A risk management approach for reducing coding and billing errors. *Journal of the National Medical Association*. 94(6): 430–447.

Bachman, J.W. 2003. The patient-computer interview: A neglected tool that can aid the clinician. *Mayo Clinic Proceedings*. 78(1): 67.

Beers, M., ed. 2006. *The Merck Manual of Diagnosis and Therapy, 18th Edition*. Whitehouse Station, NJ: Merck Research Laboratories.

Carroll, A.E., P. Tarczy-Hornoch, E. O'Reilly, and D.A. Christakis. 2003. Resident documentation discrepancies in a neonatal intensive care unit. *Journal of Pediatric Medicine*. 111(5):976.

Cascio, B. M., J. H. Wilkens, M. C. Ain, C. Toulson, and F. J. Frassica. 2005. Documentation of acute compartment syndrome at an academic healthcare center. *Journal of Bone and Joint Surgery*. 87 (2):346.

Devon, H.A. 2004. Is the medical record an accurate reflection of patients' symptoms during acute myocardial infarction? *Western Journal of Nursing Research*. 26 (5):547.

Humphreys, T., F. S. Shofer, S. Jacobson, C. Coutifaris, and A. Stemhagen. 1992. Preformatted charts improve documentation in the emergency department. *Annals of Emergency Medicine*. 21:534.

Manfield, J.A., K.L. Dodds, T.H. Mallory, A.V. Lombardo, and J.B. Adams. (2001). Linking the orthopedic office-hospital continuum: results before and after implementation of an automated patient health history project. *Orthopedic Nursing*.20(2): 51-60.

Novitsky, Y. W., R. F. Sing, K. W. Kersher, and M. L. Griffo. 2005. Blinded evaluation of accuracy of operative reports dictated by surgical residents. *The American Surgeon*. 7(8):627.

Russo, R. 2007. Improving self-efficacy and organizational performance: Identifying the differences that may exist from educational interventions crafted to utilize two versus all four self-efficacy constructs (dissertation). Cypress, CA: Touro University International.

Russo, R. 2008. Bethlehem, PA: DJ Iber Publishing.

Russo, R., and S. Fitzgerald. 2008. Physician Clinical Documentation: Implications for Healthcare Quality and Cost. Academy of Management Annual Meeting. Anaheim, CA.

Simpson, J., and E. Weiner, eds. 2005. *Oxford English Dictionary,* 6th edition. Oxford, England: Oxford University Press.

Spencer, E., T. Swanson, W. J. Hueston, and D. L. Edberg. 1999. Tools to improve documentation of smoking status: Continuous quality improvement and electronic medical records. *Archives of Family Medicine*. 8(1): 18.

Stengal, D., K. Bauwens, M. Walter, T. Kopfer, and A. Ekkerkamp. 2004. Comparison of handheld computer assisted and conventional paper chart documentation of medical records: A randomized, controlled trial. *Journal of Bone and Joint Surgery.* 86(3):553.

Timmermans, S., and M. Berg. 2003. *The Gold Standard: The Challenge of Evidence-Based Medicine and Standardization in Health Care.* Philadelphia: Temple University Press.

Weitzel, M. H., and P. R. Waller. 1990. Predictive factors for health-promotive behaviors in white, hispanic, and black blue-collar workers. *Family Community Health.* 13(1): 2334.

Chapter 2
Types of Clinical Documentation

Sources of Clinical Documentation

The sources of clinical documentation vary by type of healthcare provider organization and author of the documentation. Although physicians' entries are the primary documentation for coding and data purposes, the criteria for high-quality clinical documentation apply equally to every clinical documentation entry in every healthcare setting. The gold standard for clinical documentation in a patient record, as noted in chapter 1, is a document where all entries are legible, reliable, precise, complete, consistent, clear, and timely (AHIMA 2006; Joint Commission 2007; 42 CFR 3). This chapter describes different types of health record entries, as well as the types of provider settings where high-quality clinical documentation should be the standard. In addition, this chapter explores the priorities and focused efforts given to clinical documentation by providers in the inpatient acute care setting.

Clinical Documentation Entries

Each clinical entry in a patient's health record must meet all of the seven criteria (the gold standard) for high-quality clinical documentation. The research teams described in the summary of peer-reviewed research in chapter 1 selected discrete health record entries for their research. For example, several teams studied the completeness and quality of history and physicals, others studied progress notes, while still others focused on the problem list or operative notes. In every type of health record entry studied, researchers found significant problems with the quality of the clinical documentation.

Specific documentation responsibilities and contents of patient health records are determined by each hospital's medical staff bylaws and health records committee. However, the general contents are fundamentally the same. The most common types of entries and forms in patient health records are described along with comments about specific documentation quality concerns. It is essential to apply the criteria equally to all healthcare practitioners. Therefore, the type of author, physician or nonphysician, is also noted.

Discharge Summary

The discharge summary is a concise synopsis of the patient's course in the hospital (Huffman 1994). The biggest challenge with the discharge summary is timeliness. Although house staff or midlevel practitioners may compose or dictate the contents of a patient's discharge summary, the attending physician is the ultimate author of the discharge summary and must sign off on it accordingly (42 CFR 3). Many hospitals claim that codes are assigned to patient's record if a discharge summary is not completed in a timely manner (Russo 2001). The remedy for this lack of timeliness is to add an additional coding review for every record after the discharge summary has been completed. This requires the use of additional resources by the hospital. Discharge summaries may be inconsistent with other entries in the health record, and this necessitates the use of physician queries. Lack of clarity can also be a problem, particularly if the physician documents symptoms without identifying the etiology. At a minimum, if the cause of a symptom is not known, the physician should document the diagnosis as such. Finally, consistency may be another deficiency if the discharge summary contains information that is not supported elsewhere in the record. This may require additional communication between the coding staff and the physician (AHIMA 2008).

Problem List

The problem list can be created by a member of the house staff or a midlevel practitioner, but again, the ultimate responsibility for its contents remains with the attending physician. Problem lists are not required in all healthcare organizations, but if they are, they must be reliable. Documentation in a problem list that is inconsistent with entries in the patients' record make the list unreliable and, more importantly, it can result in quality of care concerns for the patient.

History and Physical

The patient's history and physical contains documentation that the physician uses to establish a tentative provisional diagnosis that will be the basis for treatment (Huffman 1994). Information for the history and physical report may be taken and documented by house staff or midlevel practitioners, but the attending physician has signature and ultimate responsibility for the quality of this document (42 CFR 412.46). Timeliness and legibility of the history and physical are essential because all of the clinicians treating the patient rely upon its content. Other criteria that may be an issue in the history and physical include clarity and completeness. If the author of the history and physical knows or believes a diagnosis to be present, it should be documented. If the diagnoses are differential, ruled out, probable or possible, or not established at the time of the writing, the author should document this as well.

Progress Notes

Progress notes are statements that describe the course of the patient's illness, response to treatment and status at discharge (Huffman 1994). Progress notes are documented by all physicians and clinicians treating a patient. Today, most progress notes are integrated in the health record so that caregivers can reference the progress notes of other caregivers before and after their own entries. Primary concerns about the quality of documentation in progress notes include legibility, precision, clarity, and timeliness.

Consultation Reports

Consultation reports, which contain an opinion about a patient's condition, are created by physician specialists in response to a request from the patient's attending physician (Huffman 1994). In the inpatient setting, the reports are usually dictated into a standard format designed by each hospital. In the outpatient or physician office setting, the reports are provided in a letter format from the consulting physician to the requesting physician. Regardless of the format, all consultations must meet the seven criteria for high-quality clinical documentation. The reason for most consultation requests is a search for clarity and precision in a patient's diagnosis. Therefore, these two criteria are the most essential components in consultation documentation.

Diagnostic Test Results

Diagnostic test results include radiology, cardiac, neurology, and nuclear medicine reports, among others. These test results are dictated into a report format by the physician specialist. Diagnostic test results are viewed as just one component of the patient's diagnostic process. While one test may be definitive for some patients, for most patients the combination of several tests, physician interviews and observation, and consultations are necessary pieces of the diagnostic puzzle. Clarity, reliability, and precision are of particular importance in the documentation of diagnostic tests.

Physician Orders

Orders are the physician's direction to nursing, ancillary and house staff regarding treatment for the patient (Huffman 1994). Orders may include treatment, tests, or medication. Today, many hospitals use computerized provider order entry systems (CPOEs) to ensure accuracy and reliability of the orders. For organizations that still use manual systems, physicians can enter orders themselves, but most physicians give verbal or telephone orders to a member of the nursing staff. Documentation concerns include completeness, or the inclusion of a diagnosis and/or reason for the test, medication, or other treatment being ordered.

Anesthesiology Record

The anesthesiology record is often a template that is completed by the anesthesiologist, midlevel practitioners, and nursing staff. Diagnostic information that should be recorded on the forms includes any chronic conditions the patient has, as well as any acute problems that have occurred during the current visit or during the surgery itself. Although the anesthesiologists may not be aware of this, the level of detail they document regarding the patient's diagnoses can have a significant impact on quality of care, research, and reimbursement. Completeness and precision are two documentation criteria that may not be met for anesthesiology documentation unless the providers are trained appropriately.

Operative Reports

Complete documentation for a surgical procedure includes operative progress notes and an operative report. Operative notes are documented in the patient record immediately before and after the surgery by the surgeon. The complete operative report is dictated within 24 hours of the procedure by the surgeon or a house staff member who assisted in the surgery (42 CFR 412.46; Joint Commission 2007). The attending surgeon must sign the operative report. Common problems with operative notes are legibility, clarity, and precision. Problems with the operative report may be timeliness as well as consistency, especially when the surgeon's diagnosis does not agree with the pathologist's diagnosis in the case of a surgery where tissue was removed (Cascio et al. 2005, 136).

Authors of Clinical Documentation

The criteria for high-quality clinical documentation should be applied consistently to all clinical documentation entries in all patient health records. Because it is impossible to hold anyone to a standard they are not informed about, all authors of clinical documentation should be familiar with the criteria for high-quality clinical documentation. The physician is the ultimate arbiter of the patient's care, and the physician's documentation carries a higher weight than that of other clinicians who are treating that patient (42 CFR 412.46). However, as described in the criteria for high-quality clinical documentation, the ultimate goal of all documentation in the patient's record, regardless of the author, should be to meet all of the criteria. In essence, the healthcare practitioner's documentation entries should support the other documentation in the record. This outcome is the one most likely to produce high-quality care for the patient, which is the ultimate goal of all clinical documentation practice. It is important that all individuals who document in patient records be informed about and be expected to meet clinical documentation standards.

Physician Clinical Documentation Authors

The following section describes the physician authors of clinical documentation.

Attending Physicians

Attending physicians are responsible for reviewing, approving, and signing all reports created by house staff on their behalf—generally the history and physical, the discharge summary, and the operative reports. In a nonteaching setting, the attending physician is responsible for original authorship of these documents. Attending physicians document daily progress notes and orders for the patient. In addition, attending physicians are responsible for the documentation that supports the final diagnostic statement for the patient (42 CFR 412.46). Therefore, if there is any inconsistency among different physicians who are treating a patient, the coding professionals or CDI professionals will ask the attending physician to provide the final documented response.

Consultants

Physician specialists can be asked by the attending physician to act as consultants for a patient case. Under these circumstances, the physician consultant is responsible for documenting and authenticating the consultation report. If the consultant is asked to continue to follow the patient, the consultant is responsible for documenting progress notes in the patient's record.

House Staff

House staff physicians, also known as interns, residents, and fellows, are the only treating physicians with lesser accountability because they cannot, at least in the inpatient setting, serve as attending physicians. House staff members do, however, have the same level of responsibility for consistently documenting with high-quality clinical documentation criteria. House staff physicians often have primary responsibility for documenting the history and physical, operative reports (for surgical house staff), and the discharge summary on behalf of the attending physician. They are also responsible for documenting a progress note for each patient visit that they conduct.

Surgeons

If a patient undergoes surgery during the hospital visit, the patient will have an attending surgeon. That surgeon, often referred to as the primary surgeon is responsible for documenting the pre- and post-operative progress notes as well as the operative report. In a teaching hospital, a surgical house staff member who assists during surgery will usually dictate the operative report. The attending surgeon is responsible for reviewing, approving, and signing the report. Sometimes, the attending surgeon will also be the attending physician for the patient. In this case, the surgeon has the same responsibility and accountability for documentation as the attending physician. In other instances, the patient is admitted by a primary care physician, hospitalist, or other medical specialist who serves as the patient's attending physician, and the surgeon's documentation responsibilities and accountability are limited to the surgical care of the patient.

Diagnosticians

Diagnosticians are typically not involved in the direct treatment of a patient. These professionals include radiologists, nuclear medicine physicians, and other diagnostic specialists whose primary role is to review films and test results of patients, interpret the information, and provide a diagnosis. In this role, the diagnostician's primary documentation responsibility is to document the test results and provide a diagnosis consistent with the criteria for high-quality clinical documentation. Diagnosticians' documentation cannot be relied upon solely for diagnostic coding purposes because they are not treating physicians. There must be corroboration from a treating physician, such as the attending or consultant physician. If diagnosticians become involved in direct patient care, they are held to the same level of documentation responsibility and accountability as consulting physicians.

Physician Executives

Physician executives in hospitals may or may not continue with their role as a patient-care provider. When physician executives admit and treat patients, the documentation responsibilities are consistent with those described in the section on attending physician documentation. Many physician executives serve as the physician leader for their hospital's clinical documentation program. If physician executives are also admitting or treating patients, they can serve as an example to their fellow physicians on how to practice high-quality clinical documentation. However, it is imperative that physician executives limit their documentation to only those patients they are treating. Although physician executives, in their role as clinical documentation leaders, may be reviewing the records of fellow physicians and querying physicians when the records do not meet the criteria for high-quality clinical documentation, it is important that the executive not engage in certain activities. In particular, physician executives may not tell or ask a treating physician to document something specifically in the patient's record. Physician executives can ask open-ended questions that are based on the criteria.

Nonphysician Practitioners

The following section describes the types of nonphysician practitioners who may be authors of clinical documentation.

Midlevel Practitioners

Midlevel practitioners (MLP), which include nurse practitioners and physician assistants, play an important role in delivery of care as well as supporting physicians in delivery of care. The extent of the MLP's independent activities depends on each state's laws, but in general, most states require physician supervision of the MLP. Because of the important role midlevel practitioners play in patient care, their training in clinical documentation is an essential part of an organization's clinical documentation program.

Nurses

Nurses document more frequently in a patient's health record than any other caregiver (Devon 2004). Much of the nurse's documentation involves recording data such as body temperature, input and output, and other objective and subjective indicators of the patient's current status. Nurses enter progress notes, usually in integrated progress notes with other caregivers. They review the patient's entire record frequently and are aware of all activity involving the patient. Nurses may be in one of the best positions to identify problems with deficiencies in clinical documentation. However, the nurse's responsibilities need to be focused on giving care to the patient. In addition, because the nurse documents in the patient's record, it would be impossible for the same nurse to assess the clinical documentation. Because of their unique position in giving care and providing clinical documentation, nurses should be trained in the principles of clinical documentation.

Nutritionists

Even healthcare professionals may not know that, on average, about 20 percent of all patients receive consultations from nutritionists during their hospital stay. These are, in general, the more complex cases (Hakel-Smith and Lewis 2004). Nutrition staff members have a unique opportunity to document patient nutritional and metabolic disorders with great precision. However, unless they are trained in the principles of high-quality clinical documentation, they, too, are likely to document a patient with malnutrition instead of severe protein calorie malnutrition or some other more precise diagnosis that represents the patient's condition. While a nutritionist's documentation cannot be used to translate patient health record documentation into coded data, it can be used to ask a physician for further clarification if the clinical evidence supports a more precise diagnosis.

Therapists

The list of therapists in every healthcare organization is quite long, and, depending on the patient's condition, different therapists play essential roles in the healing process. All therapists who care for patients should be identified and trained in the principles of clinical documentation. Like nutritionists, therapists (such as respiratory, physical, and occupational) have an opportunity to document the patient's condition in a precise manner. But, unless therapists are trained in the principles of clinical documentation, they are unlikely to document in a manner that consistently results in high-quality clinical documentation.

Complimentary and Integrative Practitioners

Many hospitals employ complimentary and integrative medicine (CIM) practitioners. These may include acupuncturists, naturopathic doctors, and chiropractors, among others. Like consultants, they can only treat the patient if the attending physician has requested their participation in the form of an order. CIM practitioners are responsible minimally for documenting progress notes to detail the care provided to the patient. They also may be asked to provide an initial consult and assessment, in which case they will document a report of their findings and recommendations, similar to the report of a consultant. These practitioners have the same responsibility and accountability for documentation as other caregivers, and they must meet the criteria for high-quality clinical documentation.

All Other Caregivers

When the healthcare organization performs an audit of a random sampling of its patient records, it should be able to identify all individuals who document in the patient record. These caregivers should be held to the same standards as previously described.

A Preference for the Inpatient Acute Care Setting

Because the most significant *amount* of clinical documentation per patient occurs in the inpatient setting, many organizations confine their clinical documentation program focus to inpatient records. And, in fact, this practice is supported by the peer-reviewed research described in chapter 1. However, clinical documentation and its impact permeates every patient-care setting. In fact, most healthcare in the United States occurs in the outpatient setting (Middleton and Hing 2006). Approximately 1.1 *billion* outpatient visits occur each year in the U.S. compared to approximately 35 *million* inpatient visits to acute care hospitals. Physician visits comprise about 80 percent of all outpatient visits. In all cases, but particularly when a healthcare system employs or owns physician groups, the importance of high-quality clinical documentation in every setting is clear.

Outpatient Characteristics that Impact Documentation and Coding

The following characteristics of outpatient encounters drive documentation, coding and billing practices and should be considered by every healthcare provider when designing a system to improve practices.

Different Systems for Coding and Billing

The guidelines for coding applied in the outpatient setting are different from those applied in the inpatient setting. This is relevant because the use of documentation from different providers actually varies as a result of differences in coding guidelines. Because of the volume and briefness of outpatient visits, the level of uncertainty and lack of clarity is greatly increased in the outpatient setting. This fact alone requires a high degree of proactivity from both the management and clinical teams to ensure accurate and timely documentation.

Documentation and Bill Rejection

Medical necessity plays an important role in the determination of whether a claim for outpatient care is paid at all. Medical necessity is built upon the relationship between the patient's documented diagnosis and the patient's procedure or test. Education of physicians on the appropriate way to document a patient's diagnosis can have a significant impact on the hospital's ability to bill for outpatient visits with no rejections. This one activity can require significant initial training efforts. However, it can also have a positive impact on bills being paid with no rejections.

Limited Supply of Outpatient Coding Experts

One of the best investments any healthcare organization can make is to identify and continue to cultivate internal outpatient coding experts, the individuals who translate the documentation in outpatient records into coded data. There has been a limited supply of coding professionals in the U.S. since the inception of the inpatient prospective payment system in 1982 when, suddenly, payment for inpatient services was driven by the codes assigned to the care provided to the patient. At that point, most hospitals focused their coding resources on inpatient cases. In most hospitals, the focus on ensuring that inpatient cases are accurately coded on a timely basis has continued to be the top priority, sometimes at the expense of outpatient encounters. For example, many hospitals assign the less experienced coding professional to code outpatient cases. The logic of this strategy is questionable since the numbers and complexities of guidelines, rules, and other regulatory requirements for the documentation, coding, and billing of outpatient care are much more intricate than they are for the inpatient component.

Brief Encounters

For the above reason alone, a healthcare organization might first implement the electronic health record in its outpatient setting: the average length of stay for inpatient cases is five days and the amount of time spent with an outpatient case can vary from a few minutes (a lab test) to 23 hours (observation cases) (DOH-WA 2008). The nature of the outpatient setting means that the physician or clinician must make every minute count when it comes to recording the activity involved in the patient's care during an outpatient visit. In addition, in most instances, the provider needs to make sure that documentation provided *before* the encounter is accurate and complete. This is especially true in the case of laboratory tests and other diagnostic tests. Finally, because the outpatient record is so brief, there is a tendency for physicians to rush through the documentation in such a way that often, none of the record is legible, which makes the electronic health record even more attractive to implement in this environment.

Limited Documentation and Content of the Health Records

Because of the high numbers and quick timing of outpatient visits, the amount of documentation that appears in the patient's health record, especially from physicians, is very limited for the outpatient visit. In addition, chances are very great that a healthcare organization will not be able to influence physicians to increase the amount of documentation they provide in the patient's record. It is important to create the most efficient systems for collection of outpatient documentation. The most popular strategy is to implement an electronic health record. Most of these systems allow physicians to "point and click" their way through a patient encounter, which can create additional compliance risks for the organization. The ease and efficiency of the electronic health record may result in scenarios where, for example, all boxes are automatically checked (or not checked) in a patient's history and physical report. The healthcare organization must therefore implement processes that include training and auditing to counter these possible risks.

Developing Strategies for Documentation in all Patient Settings

Whether the organization is embarking on a new clinical documentation program or is extending an existing program, it is essential to include documentation review in all patient settings. In most outpatient settings, the CDI professional or review team will have opportunities to align with physicians in a way that will impact the physicians' own medical practices. As long as the focus of CDI professionals is on providing information that is educational in nature to the organization's medical staff (and not in becoming involved in the practice's operations unless they own the practice), they should not need to be concerned about any antitrust issues. The depth of the programs may not be as comprehensive from setting to setting initially, but all settings should be included in some way. Examples of patient-care settings in which healthcare organizations will want to embrace high-quality clinical documentation include the following.

Clinical Documentation in Inpatient Settings:

- Acute care
- Subacute care
- Rehabilitation
- Skilled nursing facility
- Psychiatric hospital

Clinical Documentation in Outpatient Provider Settings:

- Physician office
- Clinic
- Same-day surgery
- Outpatient rehabilitation center
- Emergency department
- Urgent care center
- Hospital outpatient department

- Radiology and MRI center
- Diagnostic laboratory

Today, most healthcare providers have begun to align themselves and create some level of integration. For example, a *system* may include more than one hospital, several physician practices, clinics, MRI centers, a rehabilitation center, and a skilled nursing facility. Integrated healthcare systems all have their own challenges, but they have at least three things in common. They:

1. Serve patients
2. Rely on physicians to admit patients
3. Can use clinical documentation to align interests of all

Conclusion

The criteria for high-quality clinical documentation apply equally to all healthcare providers and in all healthcare settings. The gold standard for clinical documentation in a patient record is documentation that is reliable, precise, complete, consistent, clear, and timely. While different providers may have different documentation responsibilities and different levels of accountability for the portions of the health record they complete, all providers are responsible and should be held accountable for the same level of quality in their documentation. Finally, although it is tempting to focus efforts to improve documentation only in the inpatient setting, all healthcare organizations should have a plan that takes the practice into every setting including all outpatient, long-term care, and physician office locations.

References

42 CFR 412.46. 2001.

42 CFR 3. 2007. Medicare Conditions of Participation.

AHIMA. 2008. Managing an effective query process. *Journal of AHIMA* 79(10): 83–88.

Cascio, B. M., J. H. Wilkens, M. C. Ain, C. Toulson, and F. J. Frassica. 2005. Documentation of acute compartment syndrome at an academic healthcare center. *Journal of Bone and Joint Surgery*. 87(2):346.

Devon, H.A. 2004. Is the medical record an accurate reflection of patients' symptoms during acute myocardial infarction? *Western Journal of Nursing Research*. 26(5):547.

Hakel-Smith, N. and N. M Lewis. 2004. Standardized nutrition care process and language are essential components of a conceptual model to guide and document nutrition care and patient outcomes. *Journal of the American Dietetic Association*. 104(12):1878–1884.

Huffman, E.K. 1994. *Health Information Management*. Berwyn, IL: Physicians Record Company.

The Joint Commission. 2007. *Comprehensive Accreditation Manual for Hospitals, the Official Handbook*. Chicago: Joint Commission Resources.

Middleton, K. R., and E. Hing. 2006. National Hospital Ambulatory Medical Care Survey: 2004 outpatient department summary. Advance Data from Vital and Health Statistics. No. 373.

Russo, R. 2001. *National Inpatient Coder Survey*. Bethlehem, PA: HP3 Research Institute.

Washington State Department of Health (DOH-WA). 2008. Center for Health Statistics-Hospital Data. http://www.doh.wa.gov/ehsphl/hospdata/chars.htm.

Chapter 3
The Translation of Clinical Documentation into Coded Data

The Coding Process

Coding is the act of translating physician clinical documentation into diagnostic and procedural coded data. It is essentially another language, a language that allows the diagnostic, treatment, and response information of the patient to be aggregated into a uniform data set. This efficient aggregation of millions of pages of clinical documentation enables the analysis of health record information for research, planning, billing, and patient-care purposes. Without the coding professional applying a specific set of specialized skills and expertise to arrive at the coded data set for each patient, this analysis would not be possible. The coding professional needs high-quality clinical documentation to create quality data. Like the artist whose sculpture will excel if created with superior clay, so the coding professional's data product will be of higher accuracy and quality if created from superior clinical documentation.

How a Coding Professional Views an Inpatient Health Record

Within about 48 hours of being discharged from the hospital, a patient's health record is in the hands of a hospital coding professional. The coding professional is definitely the first, and may be the only person ever to read the complete health record from front to back, and this may be the first time all of the record is (or should be) in one place. It is the coding professional's job to methodically review all of the information in the record so the clinical documentation can be translated into the language of coding. The next few paragraphs contain a description of the steps a typical coding professional is likely to take in reviewing a patient health record for coding purposes. The exact order of review may vary by coding professional or by the way a record, especially an electronic health record, is compiled. The coding professional begins the review with the first page of the record, which is commonly known as the *face sheet* or the *admission and discharge form*. The face sheet is a summary piece of paper that contains primarily demographic information. Usually the upper half of the page contains the patient's demographic and insurance information. A coding professional may take note of the patient's age and the admission and discharge dates, which are also on the form and then do a quick calculation to determine how long the patient was in the hospital by subtracting the admission date from the discharge date. These two pieces of information give the coding professional a basic idea of the complexity of the record. For example, the record of an 89-year-old patient in the hospital for nine days would be more complex to review and code than the record of a 29-year-old who was in and out of the hospital within two days. Of course, another simple and obvious clue to the complexity is the size of the patient's record. Usually, the thicker the record, the more complex the case was. The lower half of the face sheet is a blank space where the physician documents the patient's diagnoses and procedures. This documentation may be fairly sketchy, but it gives the coding professional some initial clues about what was going on with the patient.

The next form in the patient's record is usually the discharge summary, if it was completed by the physician immediately after discharge. The discharge summary, which should provide a complete overview of the patient's entire stay, is generally the last document completed for the patient's record. The next document that appears in the record, the history and physical, is the first document completed during the patient's stay. Coding professionals read the complete history and physical, and they look for key pieces of information. Things like symptoms upon admission, medications that the patient was taking, and chronic conditions are important to note. The attending physician's "impression and plan", which usually appears at the end of the history and physical, helps the coding professional to piece together the patient's diagnoses.

The next stack of pages in the patient's record contains the progress notes. For a coding professional, the progress notes are the essence of the patient's record. Reading and deciphering the progress notes, which are almost always handwritten, can be challenging. The notes represent what was going on in the physician's mind at that point in time. There is something about the candidness of the progress notes that cannot be captured in a dictated and transcribed formal report. The day-by-day description of treatment activities and the patient's reactions to treatment versus reading the discharge summary is like the difference between watching the news happen versus listening to it being delivered on television that night.

Consultation reports are typically the next set of documents in a patient's record. Consultation reports are particularly important for coding professionals. When coding professionals review the consultation report, they try to determine whether the attending physician and the consultant were in agreement with each other on the patient's diagnosis. If not, the coding professional may need to contact the attending physician to clarify the patient's diagnosis. If one physician documents that the patient had a stroke and another physician documents that the same patient had a TIA, the coding professional needs a tie breaker; and the attending, or primary, physician breaks the tie in every case. When a documentation discrepancy between the attending and another treating physician occurs, the coding professional generates a query to the attending physician to clarify the patient's diagnosis and resolve the conflicting documentation in the patient's record.

Diagnostic test results are the next set of documents reviewed by coding professionals. Diagnostic test results present some of the biggest challenges for hospital coding professionals. In fact, the codes that some coding professionals assigned based on abnormal diagnostic test results alone came under so much scrutiny by the federal government in the mid-1990s that hospitals were fined over $2 billion in 1997. The activity for codes being assigned based upon abnormal test results only (without adequate documentation by the physician) is commonly known as assumption coding and is in violation of federal regulations and statutory law. Today, the guidelines for what coding professionals do with abnormal test results are much clearer than they were in 1997. Abnormal test results without a physician verification of a diagnosis or documentation as to whether the test result is clinically-significant prompts the coding professional to query the physician. If the physician documents the diagnosis, then the coding professional can translate that documentation into a code. If the physician does not document the diagnosis, the coding professional cannot assume the patient has a diagnosis based

Figure 3.1   Required documentation for the coding of abnormal laboratory tests

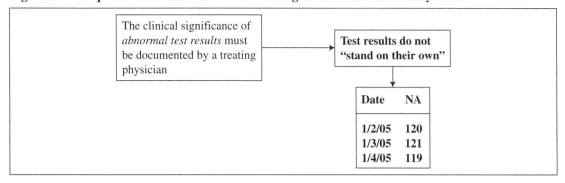

Figure 3.2   Required documentation for coding from physician orders

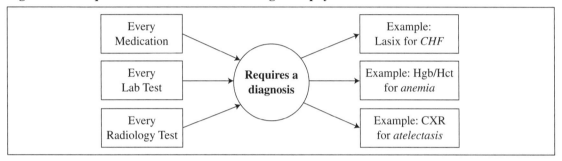

solely on abnormal test results. Figures 3.1 and 3.2 illustrate the required documentation from the physician that a coding professional needs to use clinical information such as abnormal lab results, orders, or medication administration records for coding purposes.

If a patient has surgery performed during the hospital stay, the next set of forms in the record will be the surgical suite of forms: the preoperative or preanesthesia assessment completed by the anesthesiologist; a formal operative report completed by the surgeon; a postoperative assessment completed by the anesthesiologist; and, if any tissue was removed during the surgery, a pathology report completed by the hospital pathologist. Coding professionals read the surgical report very closely to determine exactly what surgeries were performed that need to be coded. In addition, anesthesiologists often document patient conditions that might not be documented by other physicians who are treating the patient. This is particularly true of chronic respiratory conditions or heart murmurs that may be significant for the anesthesiologist to monitor while the patient is under anesthesia. Any information documented by the anesthesiologist that conflicts with that of the attending physician may require a query to the attending physician.

Physician orders are the next part of the patient record. Coding professionals check to make sure that they have been able to assign a diagnostic code to the reason for every order placed. For example, if the physician places an order on a record for Lasix, a drug used to treat congestive heart failure (CHF), but there is no documentation for congestive heart failure on the record, this may trigger a question from the coding professional to the physician to clarify the diagnoses.

Nurses' graphic records appear after physician orders in the patient record. One of the common items coding professionals look for here is the patient's temperature. If a nurse charted a high temperature and the patient was treated with antibiotics or analgesics, coding professionals want to make sure there is a corresponding diagnosis documented by the physician for this activity. Coding professionals are always looking to close the loop and make sure that the activities in the record match with the diagnoses. Closing the loop means that the codes present an accurate picture of what actually happened to the patient during the stay.

Finally, medication administration forms appear in the record. Many coding professionals first review the medication administration forms. By looking at these forms, coding professionals can quickly get an idea of what is wrong with the patient. The medications or intravenous (IV) fluids that were administered to the patient during the stay provide good evidence of what happened. So, a coding professional may begin with a hypothesis such as: the patient received antibiotics, Lasix, and potassium in his or her IV fluids, therefore, the patient probably had an infection (treated with antibiotics), CHF (treated with Lasix), and low potassium, also known as hypokalemia (treated with potassium supplements). Next, the coding professional begins at the front of the record looking for evidence to support the hypothesis. Of course, coding professionals identify other information while wading through the record, but using the medication administration forms to formulate a hypothesis can be quite reliable.

The Relationship between Clinical Documentation and Coding

The coding professional's job includes:

1. Reviewing all clinical documentation in the patient's record

2. Separating out clinical information that has been documented with high quality by the physician into diagnoses for coding purposes

3. Applying rules for "whose documentation counts" for coding purposes

4. Including only diagnoses and procedures that should be coded under official coding guidelines

5. Arriving at the correct code number to represent the diagnosis or procedure (CMS and NCHS 2006)

6. Asking the physician about any gaps in documentation that may represent a diagnosis that is clinically but not sufficiently documented. The preferred methodology for physician querying is concurrent, while the patient is still in-house, as illustrated in figure 3.3. However, when a query cannot be asked concurrently due to a short length-of-stay or the physician does not respond, the coding professional is charged with asking the physician to clarify any documentation which was authored that does not meet high-quality clinical documentation criteria (AHIMA 2008).

Basic Coding Guidelines

All codes are assigned using the official ICD-9-CM coding manuals. These manuals contain directions for coding professionals to use when assigning codes. However, in the instance when a coding professional encounters an issue that is not addressed in the manual, the Centers for Medicare and Medicaid Services (CMS) and the National Center for Health Statistics (NCHS), two departments within the Department of Health and Human Services (HHS), have created the *ICD-9-CM Official Guidelines for Coding and Reporting* (CMS and NCHS 2006).

Figure 3.3   Methodology for querying physicians

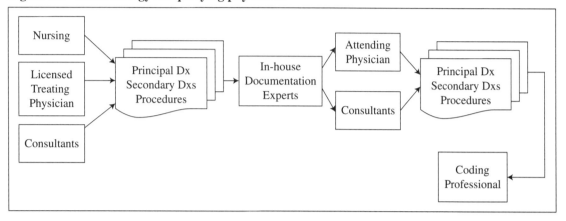

The guidelines were developed and approved by the cooperating parties for ICD-9-CM. The cooperating parties are the American Hospital Association (AHA), the American Health Information Management Association (AHIMA), CMS, and the NCHS (CMS and NCHS 2006). The first paragraph of the guidelines contains the following sentence: "A joint effort between the attending physician and coder is essential to achieve complete and accurate documentation, code assignment, and reporting of diagnoses and procedures." This statement further emphasizes the importance of high-quality clinical documentation as well as the role of the coding professional in assuring the final coded data is consistent with the documentation in the patient's record. Detailed information can be obtained from the guidelines, but the two most important and basic definitions are for the assignment of a patient's principal diagnosis and for the secondary diagnoses in the inpatient setting. The definitions are the following:

Principal diagnosis: Every inpatient is assigned one principal ICD-9-CM diagnostic code. The principal diagnosis is the condition that is determined, after study, to have caused the admission of the patient to the acute care setting *and* is documented by a licensed, treating physician.

Secondary diagnosis: Every inpatient is assigned one ICD-9-CM diagnostic code for every diagnosis that is documented by a licensed, treating physician, and is either clinically evaluated, treated, and tested during the stay or responsible for increasing the length of stay or use of resources (CMS and NCHS 2006).

Another way to view the patient's principal and secondary diagnoses is illustrated in table 3.1. This table shows the differences between acute and chronic conditions as well as the importance of precision and completeness in all clinical documentation for diagnoses.

Example of Coding for a Myocardial Infarction (Heart Attack)

The following example provides some insight into the detail involved in coding a patient's diagnosis. A coding professional needs to be adept at reading the entire health record. Then, the individual must be able to translate the material, through his or her expertise and a series of filters, into the representative codes. Table 3.2 presents a list that includes all the different codes available for patients who are admitted to the hospital with a current, acute myocardial infarction (MI) or heart attack. There are additional codes for patients who have had the MI prior to hospital admission, or in situations where the physician has not documented exactly when the heart attack occurred.

Table 3.1   Clinical documentation characteristics

Important Considerations	Document . . .	Examples: If present or suspected, document . . .
Patient's principal diagnosis	Detail, precision	*"Aspiration"* pneumonia *"Acute"* renal failure Cerebral *"infarct"*
Chronic coexisting diagnoses	Everything under consideration	COPD CHF Seizure disorder Pulmonary fibrosis
Acute coexisting diagnoses	Everything being evaluated or treated	Malnutrition, Respiratory failure Dehydration
Abnormal diagnostic tests	The clinical significance of	Hyponatremia Mitral regurgitation Atrial fibrillation
Symptoms	The etiology or "suspected etiology"	Instead of Chest pain—Possible GERD Angina due to CAD Instead of Syncope—Arrhythmia

Table 3.2   Examples of the use of the fifth digit for coding

Code	Condition
410.01	[MI/heart attack] of the anteriolateral wall
410.11	[MI/heart attack] of other anterior wall (i.e. anterioapical or anteroseptal wall)
410.21	[MI/heart attack] of the inferolateral wall
410.31	[MI/heart attack] of the interoposterior wall
410.41	[MI/heart attack] of other interior wall (i.e., diaphragmatic wall)
410.51	[MI/heart attack] of other lateral wall (i.e., basal-lateral, high lateral)
410.61	[MI/heart attack] of the true posterior wall
410.71	[MI/heart attack] of the subendocardium (also nontransmural infarct)
410.81	[MI/heart attack] of other specified sites (i.e., atrium, papillary muscle)
410.91	[MI/heart attack] of unspecified site of heart

Each code designates very specific information. The digits to the left of the decimal represent the main condition (MI or heart attack). The digits to the right are based upon the specific location and timing of the patient's heart attack. Examples in table 3.2 using the fifth digit "1" show that the MI occurred during the current admission. Other fifth digits are available to identify that an MI occurred during a prior admission (414.02) or that an MI occurred neither during the current nor a prior admission (414.00). The use of a fifth digit 0 or 2, particularly, would be a red flag to identify that the physician's clinical documentation does not meet the criteria for high-quality clinical documentation. The coding professional, especially in the inpatient setting, should always be able to determine, based upon the physician's documentation, whether an MI occurred during the current or a prior admission (ICD-9-CM 2007).

The details used in codes in the ICD-9-CM coding book are generally to facilitate medical research. For example, certain areas of the heart affected by heart attacks may respond better to certain drugs or interventions than others. However, if coding professionals grouped all patients' heart attacks together under one general code, there would be no way of comparing large data bases of patients with heart attacks as researchers do today.

Insurance companies and Medicare also use the detailed ICD-9-CM coding to determine if the information is sufficient for them to pay the bill. Certain insurance companies and Medicare may reject codes that are "unspecified." For example, the heart attack code 410.90 represents "heart attack of unspecified site of the heart, unspecified as to episode of care." If this code is submitted on a patient's bill, it could be a red flag for an insurance company, and the bill could be rejected unless more detailed codes are submitted by the provider. The insurance company's perspective is that if the hospital treated the patient for a heart attack, they should know if it was a current, acute attack (a fifth digit of "1" instead of "0"), and they should probably know where in the heart muscle the blood flow was stopped.

Impacts of Documentation and Coding

Severity of Illness

Since 1982, CMS has paid for Medicare acute care hospital stays using a method of grouping ICD-9-CM codes into like categories known as diagnosis-related groups (DRGs). The original CMS DRG system, premised upon statistically significant formulas that reflect resource utilization by the hospital, assumed that under the system some patient cases will be losers (economically) and others will be winners for the hospital. Since 2008, CMS has used a more refined version of the DRG system that relies to a greater degree on a patient's severity of illness instead of just resource utilization to calculate reimbursement. Severity-based DRGs have been called the equalizer for prospective inpatient reimbursement. Severity-based DRGs seek to even the playing field by drawing upon all of the possible diagnoses, simple procedures, and treatments for a patient to create a profile for reimbursement that is clinically-significant and accurately reflects the patient's severity of illness and risk of mortality (MedPAC 2006).

Three severity-based DRG systems commonly are used to group and analyze inpatient documentation. They are Medicare Severity DRGs (MS-DRGs), All Patient Diagnosis-Related Groups (AP-DRGs), and All Patient Refined Diagnosis-Related Groups (APR-DRGs). The MS-DRGs have been in use by CMS for Medicare reimbursement since 2008. AP-DRGs, created by 3M, are used by several states for Medicaid reimbursement. APR-DRGs, also created by 3M, are used to analyze some portion of the data for Medicare Quality Indicators, and these also are used for several commercial hospital quality reporting Web-based products (Averill et al. 2003).

In addition to its economic appeal, the use of a clinically-significant measurement system, such as the severity-based DRG systems, is appealing to the physician members of the hospital community. Most physicians understand and are drawn to data that reflect clinical measures for their patients and themselves. Severity measures appear to do just that. To ensure accurate severity measures, the hospital's clinical documentation and resulting coded data must be of high quality.

Table 3.3 demonstrates the differences in DRG assignment among the MS-, AP-, and APR-DRG systems.

Present on Admission

In 2007, CMS began to require hospitals to identify secondary diagnoses that are present on admission (POA) for Medicare inpatient cases. The overall purpose of the POA indicator is to differentiate between conditions present at admission and conditions that

Table 3.3   Levels of DRGs in each system

MS-DRGs	AP-DRGs	APR DRGs
Stand alone DRGs (TIA)	Stand alone DRGs (TIA)	No stand alone DRGs
Without a CC	Without a CC	Severity 1 (minor)
With a CC	With a CC	Severity 2 (moderate)
With a Major CC	With a Major CC	Severity 3 (major)
		Severity 4 (extreme)

develop during an inpatient admission. As of 2008, the diagnoses not POA are coded, but are not included in the DRG calculation. The collection of the POA indicator for secondary diagnoses is yet another reason to implement a clinical documentation improvement program. The ultimate goal of the POA program is to craft a reimbursement system that considers not only severity and resource utilization, but also quality indicators. Essentially, diagnoses that are not POA are considered a quality concern and are not included in the calculation for payment (CMS and NCHS Supplement 2006). These diagnoses include:

- Serious preventable event, object left in surgery
- Serious preventable event, air embolism
- Serious preventable event, blood incompatibility
- Catheter-associated urinary tract infection
- Pressure ulcers (decubitus)
- Vascular catheter-associated infection
- Mediastinitis after cardiac artery bypass grafting, surgical site infection
- Hospital-acquired injuries (fracture, dislocation, intracranial injury, crushing injury, burn, and other unspecified effects of external causes)

Examples of types of documentation that might be used to determine POA assignment include emergency room notes, history and physical, and progress and admitting notes. Other documentation that can be helpful includes:

- Conditions present and diagnosed prior to admission
- Conditions diagnosed as existing during the admission process and therefore present before admission
- Any suspected, possible, probable, or to-be-ruled-out conditions
- Differential diagnoses
- Underlying causes of any sign or symptom present on admission
- Specific identification of acute or chronic status of any condition
- External causes (the "how" and "where") of injury or poisoning in the physician's notes

Coding in Settings Other Than Acute Care

ICD-9-CM coding guidelines for outpatient clinical documentation are also included in the Official Guidelines for Coding and Reporting (CMS and NCHS 2006). In outpatient settings, ICD-9-CM codes are used to assign a code to the patient's diagnoses. However, Current Procedural Terminology (CPT) codes are used to assign a code to any procedures or physician office visits (AMA 2008). CPT coding manuals are published by the American Medical Association and coding guidelines for use of the CPT manuals are also published by the AMA. Outpatient coding professionals are trained in coding for the physician office and the outpatient setting. The documentation and coding requirements for both settings are detailed and vary greatly by setting. However, the same criteria for high-quality clinical documentation in the inpatient setting also apply to the outpatient setting.

Conclusion

Coding is the act of translating physician clinical documentation into diagnostic and procedural coded data. It is essentially another language—a language that allows the diagnostic, treatment, and response information of the patient to be aggregated into a uniform data set. This efficient aggregation of millions of pages of clinical documentation enables the analysis of health record information for research, planning, billing, and patient-care purposes. High-quality clinical documentation is needed to produce high quality coded data.

It may be helpful for clinical documentation professionals and other clinicians to understand how a coding professional views a health record. Documentation professionals can use this understanding to guide their review and query process. It is also helpful for documentation professionals to understand the complexity of both the ICD-9-CM coding system and the official coding guidelines. The level of detail required in the coding system is one justification for the need for such detail in clinical documentation. Finally, it is also important to understand that coding guidelines and systems vary based on the healthcare provider setting. In particular, coding guidelines are different for the outpatient and physician office settings than they are for the hospital setting. The CPT coding system is used for coding outpatient procedures and physician office visits. Although coding systems and guidelines may be different, the criteria for high-quality clinical documentation remain consistent across all provider settings.

References

AHIMA. 2008. Managing an effective query process. *Journal of AHIMA* 79(10): 83–88.

American Medical Association. (2008). *Current Procedural Terminology*, Chicago: American Medical Association.

Averill, R. F., G. Norbert., J. S. Hughes, et al. 2003. *All Patient Refined Diagnosis Related Groups, Definitions Manual, Version 20.0*, Volumes 1, 2, and 3. Wallingford, CT: 3M Health Information Systems.

Centers for Medicare and Medicaid Services (CMS) and the National Center for Health Statistics (NCHS). 2006. *ICD-9-CM Official Guidelines for Coding and Reporting*. www.cdc.gov/nchs/datawh/ftpserv/ftpicd9/ftpicd9.htm.

Centers for Medicare and Medicaid Services (CMS) and the National Center for Health Statistics (NCHS). 2006. *ICD-9-CM Official Guidelines for Coding and Reporting—Supplement. 2006*. http://www.cdc.gov/nchs/data/icd9/POAguideSep06.pdf.

ICD-9-CM Coding Book. 2007. Government Printing Office, Washington, DC

MedPAC. 2006 (September). Payment Basics: Hospital Acute Inpatient Services Payment System. http:www.medpac.gov/publications/other-reports/Sept06_MedPAC_Payment-Basics_hospital.pdf.

Chapter 4
Assessing Clinical Documentation

The Importance of a Clinical Documentation Assessment

An assessment is a snapshot in time that gives the clinical documentation improvement (CDI) review team or CDI specialists a starting point for their activities. Unless the review team is familiar with the organization's documentation and the data that is produced from it, it cannot determine whether its efforts to improve clinical documentation have been successful. Reviewing actual documentation and data prior to investing in a CDI program prevents the CDI review team from acting on assumptions. For example, the management team may believe there is a quality problem with clinical documentation based upon discussions, a drop in case mix, and a few examples of documentation problems identified in patient records during the coding process. In this case, the organization should perform an objective analysis of both data and documentation for two reasons. First, an analysis will determine whether the perceived problem exists. Second, the analysis, if performed consistent with the recommendations in this chapter, will provide a valid baseline for measuring the impact of any CDI efforts.

If the organization already has a CDI program in place, it can use the information in this chapter to validate its current baseline. The information also can be used to determine whether current analyses include all of the necessary components. If not, then this chapter can be used to include some new baseline analytics in the process. Finally, if a program currently is in place that only focuses on inpatient documentation, then this information can be used to analyze outpatient or long-term care data and create a baseline for those care areas. In every case, it is important to include analyses of both data and documentation for any assessment.

Data Review

Every healthcare organization produces significant amounts of data on an ongoing basis. As noted in the introduction to this book, this data is used for everything from reimbursement and quality indicators to research and planning. A management team that knows, understands, and uses the data produced by its organization is more likely to make better decisions than a team that is not data-centered (Drucker 1999). The use of data for decision making is most imperative when the decisions involve a new or an established CDI program.

What Data Matters?

There are two types of data to be considered in the CDI process. The first is the data the organization itself produces. The second is the data that others produce about the organization. An organization produces data from coding, data collected for quality indicators, and other specialized data collected for the organization's mortality and morbidity review (MMR) or other internal clinical committees or groups.

An organization collects a significant amount of data that must be prioritized to focus its efforts and obtain maximum benefit from this data review. There are certain general guidelines that are included in this chapter, but data varies for each organization based on individual needs. One of the first questions to ask is what level of aggregation to look at. Many organizations want to begin at a high level and drill down to the details if a problem or unexpected finding is discovered in the high level data. For coded data, one of the highest levels of aggregation is by DRG. The organization may also want to consider reviewing data by severity level or by the presence or absence of complication and comorbidity (CC) codes. One of the most detailed levels of data is found at the diagnosis or procedure code level. Table 4.1 shows hospital severity levels from the All Patient Refined (APR) grouper broken out by service type. This shows another way to drill into high level data. The review begins with data by severity. Within each severity level, the type of service is specified. This type of data review can help determine whether there may be specific problems in certain clinical departments. In table 4.1, the orthopedic service shows 45 percent of patients with severity level 1 and only 14 percent of patients with severity level 3. These two numbers show that orthopedic patients have lower severity levels than patients in all other services. There may be a reason to expect that orthopedic patients are less severely ill than those in all other services. If not, this data finding is a red flag that orthopedic services may have a more significant problem with documentation practices than other services.

Data that others produce about the organization has an impact on patient perception, accreditation status, and reimbursement. These data include Medicare quality indicators, The Joint Commission's Quality Check, private quality organizations like HealthGrades, and state-specific quality programs like the Medisgroup data abstracting used by states like Colorado and Pennsylvania (PHCCCC 2006). An example of data produced by HealthGrades for patients to review appears in figure 4.1.

Hospitals with one star are providing care below the quality expected, those with three stars are providing care at the level of quality expected, and those with five stars are providing better quality than expected for the diagnosis or procedure analyzed. If an organization has a one- or three-star rating that it believes should be a five-star rating, documentation may be the reason. Furthermore, analysis at this level will allow comparison of ratings by service since HealthGrades provides ratings by diagnosis and by procedure.

Table 4.1. Hospital severity levels from the APR grouper based on service type

Service	Minor (Level 1)	Moderate (Level 2)	Major (Level 3)	Extreme (Level 4)
Internal Medicine	40%	32%	25%	3%
Cardiology	35%	35%	28%	2%
Neurology	30%	40%	27%	3%
General Surgery	28%	42%	25%	5%
Orthopedic Surgery	45%	40%	14%	1%

Figure 4.1   Example of hospital quality ratings by Healthgrades

Hospital's Name	Inhospital Mortality (Survival)	Inhospital +1 Month Mortality (Recovery +30)	Inhospital +6 Month Mortality (Recovery +180)	
✚ = view details	2005 Ratings Atrial Fibrillation			
High Volume Hospitals				
✚ St Lukes Hospital Newburgh, NY	★★★	★★★	★★★	
✚ St Lukes Cornwall Hospital Newburgh, NY	★★★	★★★	★★★	
✚ Good Samaritan Hospital Of Suffern Suffern, NY	★★★	★★★	★★★	
✚ Benedictine Hospital Kingston, NY	★★★	★★★	★★★	
✚ Catskill Regional Medical Center Harris, NY	★★★	★★★	★★★	
✚ Bon Secours Community Hospital Port Jervis, NY	★★★	★★★	★★★	
✚ Kingston Hospital Kingston, NY	★	★★★	★★★	
✚ Nyack Hospital Nyack, NY	★	★	★★★	
✚ Orange Regional Medical Center Goshen, NY	★★★	★	★	
✚ St Anthony Community Hospital Warwick, NY	★	★	★	

www.healthgrades.com. Used with permission.

Using Criteria to Screen the Data

Everything is relative, and a valid comparison is needed for the data. Three sources of comparative data include:

1. Normative data

2. Regulatory guidance

3. The organization's own benchmarks

National normative data can be used, but it is much more relevant to use data from hospitals that are similar in size, teaching status, and geographic status. Some organizations have their own information staff who are able to obtain detailed levels of data.

In addition, the data can be purchased for reasonable rates from organizations like the American Hospital Directory (AHD) (http://www.ahd.com/). Other sources of data may be found in the regulatory guidance provided by the Office of the Inspector General (OIG), Medicare, Quality Improvement Organizations (QIOs), and other governmental agencies. For example, on some occasions local QIOs have published complication and comorbidity rates or certain DRG pair proportions that raise a red flag for the review team (IPRO 2005a; IPRO 2005b). Finally, the organization's own benchmarks can be used to screen data (so long as this is consistent with legal and regulatory requirements). Ideally, an organization will develop its own set of criteria based upon the three sources.

Deciding What Data to Review

Once the CDI review team has decided on what criteria to use, it needs to determine what data to review. Ultimately, what the team reviews is driven by two things: the criteria used to screen the data for decision making and the purpose of the review. For example, what is the team trying to get out of the data review? For high-quality clinical documentation, one of the criteria is completeness. One way to apply the criteria to aggregate level data is to identify patient records with vague principal diagnoses. While these may be valid from a high level data perspective, a vague or symptomatic principal diagnosis can be a red flag. Table 4.2 illustrates this type of data. Medicare was separated out from other payers since the age difference may impact the data. The figure represents discharges for a 300-bed hospital over the course of a year. The hospital in this case was concerned about the high numbers of chest pain and vertigo cases. At a minimum, this type of data analysis can provide the organization with enough information to know it should explore the issue of clinical documentation quality further.

Recommended Data to Review

This section presents a list of recommended data to review. It is important, however, to ensure that the data review is reflective of the organization. This list is intended as a general guide only. Each organization should create a data review that will accomplish the organization's specific objectives.

Discharges by Service and by Major Diagnostic Category

It is important that the CDI review team understand which are the most common services admitting patients to the hospital. It is particularly important to review the data by service if the service is assigned by an indicator other than major diagnostic category (MDC). Then, discharges by service should be compared with discharges by MDC.

Table 4.2   Discharges for a 300-bed hospital during a 12-month period

Diagnosis	Medicare	Other Payors
Chest Pain	53	436
Syncope	50	166
Angina	70	250
Back pain	43	128
Vertigo	26	223
Epistaxis	12	61
Shortness of Breath	11	90
Musculoskeletal pain	10	36

www.ahd.com. Used with permission.

Lack of agreement between the two may point to a problem with clinical documentation. For example, when cardiologists are admitting a significant number of patients with chest pain to the hospital, discharges by MDC may show a lower number of cardiac admissions than discharges by service. This difference could represent a problem with precision in documenting a principal diagnosis.

Table 4.3 is an example of data about the organization that can be obtained from the American Hospital Directory (AHD 2008). This data is derived from MedPAR data, so it is usually more than a year old. It is a starting point for analysis, but ultimately, more recent data provided by the organization's internal information or finance staff will be wanted.

Discharges by DRG

Most organizations review data by DRG on a regular basis as part of their case mix analysis. For clinical documentation purposes, actual DRG data should be reviewed against the organization's expectations. For example, an organization may believe there are no (or very little) inpatient admissions for chest pain since it opened the chest pain clinic. If an analysis of DRG level data reveals several cases in the chest pain DRG, this is a red flag for documentation.

Case Mix Index

Most organizations review case mix index (CMI) over time, both overall and by specialty. For clinical documentation analysis purposes, an unexpected change in CMI could signal a possible problem with clinical documentation. For example, if the CMI for orthopedic surgery has dropped for the past six months with no change in admitting physicians or types of surgery performed, it may be that the orthopedic surgeons are not completely documenting all diagnoses in their patients' records.

Table 4.3   Examples of data that can be obtained from the American Hospital Directory

	Number Medicare Inpatients	Average Length of Stay	Average Charges	Average Cost	Medicare CMI
Burns	28	12.11	$78,359	$21,436	2.6269
Cardiology	1,925	4.79	$22,065	$6,314	1.0917
Cardiovascular Surgery	1,667	6.13	$88,352	$19,704	3.7755
Gynecology	92	3.49	$21,137	$5,505	1.1344
Medicine	3,304	4.23	$18,367	$5,159	0.8810
Neurology	977	4.56	$22,068	$6,098	1.0861
Neurosurgery	108	8.85	$67,128	$17,910	2.9322
Oncology	290	6.80	$26,945	$7,545	1.4957
Orthopedics	1,766	5.25	$31,757	$8,135	1.7000
Psychiatry	601	11.82	$21,155	$8,180	0.6840
Pulmonology	1,322	7.54	$51,775	$13,428	2.5170
Surgery	1,018	8.43	$52,132	$13,687	2.3922
Surgery for Malignancy	74	4.70	$30,470	$8,019	1.6887
Urology	812	4.85	$25,879	$8,107	1.2416
Vascular Surgery	394	6.37	$42,201	$11,444	2.0163
TOTAL	14,387	5.79	$36,259	$9,451	1.6964

www.ahd.com. Used with permission.

Complication and Major Complication Rates

Changes in rates, or rates that are not consistent with an organization's expectations or normative data, may indicate a problem with clinical documentation quality. Table 4.4 is an example of a report that shows overall CC capture rate by all medicine and all surgical specialties together and then by each specialty. The comparison with peer norms for Medicare cases is helpful in determining whether rates appear to be lower or higher than an organization's norms. Any inconsistency provides support for further clinical documentation review and analysis.

Severity Levels (MS-DRGs and APR-DRGs)

If the CDI review team has access to the MS-DRG and the APR-DRG grouper, it is helpful to look at the organization's severity levels for both groupers. While MS-DRGs are used for Medicare reimbursement, the APR-DRG grouper is used for quality indicators for HealthGrades' analysis and by many states for Medicaid reimbursement. Changes in rates or inconsistency with expectations or normative data may indicate a problem with clinical documentation quality.

Medicare Quality Indicators

Since Medicare quality indicators are important for both reimbursement (pay for performance) and accreditation (The Joint Commission uses many of the same measures), it is essential to be familiar with the organization's outcomes data. Table 4.5 contains a summary of the Medicare quality indicators for a hospital for current, reported indicators (CMS 2008). In this example, a hospital may identify that documentation of influenza and pneumococcal vaccination status may be an issue for physician documentation.

Table 4.4   Complication and comorbidity (CC) capture rates—combined and by specialty

CC Capture Rate	Medicare	Other Payers	Medicare Peer Norms
All Medicine Specialties	68%	50%	81%
All Surgical Specialties	77%	39%	72%
General Medicine	70%	50%	80%
Cardiology	79%	46%	93%
General Surgery	68%	43%	78%
Orthopedic Surgery	59%	28%	69%

Table 4.5   Example of summary of Medicare quality indicators

Measure: Pneumonia					
Condition	**# of Pts**	**Hosp Score**	**Nat'l Avg**	**90th %tile**	**State Avg**
Appropriate Initial Antibiotic Selection	140	89%	87%	97%	88%
Blood Cultures Performed in the Emergency Department Prior to Initial Antibiotic Received in Hospital	237	86%	90%	100%	90%
Influenza Vaccination Status	65	97%	75%	99%	79%
Initial Antibiotic(s) within 6 Hours After Arrival	190	93%	93%	100%	93%
Oxygenation Assessment	344	99%	99%	100%	100%
Pneumococcal Vaccination Status	310	95%	78%	97%	85%
Smoking Cessation Advice/Counseling	91	100%	85%	100%	93%

Secondary Diagnoses

The numbers of secondary diagnoses for inpatient cases can provide some insight into the level of detail of documentation available to the coding staff for code assignment. If this measure is used for CDI, the review team will want to make sure its members are familiar with the coding guidelines at the hospital and understand any possible limitations. The team may also want to delete one-day stays from the data since they can skew overall averages. Table 4.6 uses severity levels to stratify numbers of secondary diagnoses. This table reveals that the numbers of secondary diagnoses for this hospital for all cases are less than those for peer hospitals. It points in particular to a possible significant problem with surgery cases since the peer norms figure is 6.5 secondary diagnoses on average, while the hospital has only 5.6 secondary diagnoses for surgery cases. Secondary diagnoses can also be stratified by service and physician for more detail.

Data Considerations for Reviewing Outpatient Clinical Documentation

Most clinical documentation assessments seem to focus, at least initially, on inpatient documentation. However, more than 50 percent of healthcare systems' revenue is now driven by outpatient stays (AHD 2008). Therefore, outpatient clinical documentation should be included in every organization's documentation improvement initiatives. Data review opportunities for outpatient analyses are more abundant than for inpatient analyses. Part of the reason for this is that all outpatient cases cannot be reduced to 500 or so categories, such as with the DRG system that is used for inpatient cases. While there are some aggregations via the ambulatory payment classifications (APCs), one outpatient can be assigned more than one APC. Furthermore, APCs are not assigned to all outpatient cases. Therefore, in some instances, the analysis remains at the code level for some outpatients.

Organizations can create their own reporting system for outpatient analysis. The American Hospital Directory provides a Web-based resource to generate reports such as those shown in tables 4.7 and 4.8 (AHD 2008). These include:

1. Top 20 medical diagnoses

2. Top 20 APCs

3. Number of cases

4. Financial information

Table 4.6   Comparison of secondary diagnoses

Number of secondary diagnoses for:	Number	Peer Norms
All inpatient cases	5.3	6.8
Medicine cases	5.6	7.2
Surgical cases	4.2	6.6
Severity Level 1 cases	2.6	2.8
Severity Level 2 cases	5.3	5.5
Severity Level 3 cases	8.6	9.0
Severity Level 4 cases	11.8	12.0

Table 4.7   Statistics for the top 20 medical diagnoses

ICD-9 Code	ICD-9 Description	Total Payment	Number Patient Claims	Average Charge	Average Cost	Average Payment	Total Outlier Amount	National Average Charge
V580	RADIOTHERAPY ENCOUNTER	$4,122,061	1,308	$11,520	$3,461	$3,151	$18,919	$6,773
V581	CHEMOTHERAPY ENCOUNTER	$1,743,963	1,755	$6,184	$1,598	$993	$123,099	$7,359
28522	ANEMIA NEO DIS	$953,915	1,691	$3,635	$1,015	$564	$190,180	$3,159
41401	CAD	$446,410	213	$8,027	$1,840	$2,095	$790	$6,309
2859	ANEMIA NOS	$359,570	785	$2,398	$795	$458	$58,740	$1,564
1985	SEC MALIG BONE	$323,846	371	$4,052	$974	$872	$13,387	$3,114
185	MALIGN PROSTATE	$260,317	384	$2,952	$800	$677	$3,408	$3,477
2880	AGRANULOCYTOSIS	$251,534	376	$3,258	$879	$668	$31,064	$1,883
78659	CHEST PAIN NEC	$235,678	221	$4,077	$961	$1,066	$869	$2,882
V7612	SCREEN MAMMO	$228,930	3,843	$175	$33	$59	$0	$207
V6709	F/U SURGERY NEC	$226,928	707	$1,170	$342	$320	$851	$1,028
72402	SPINAL STENOSIS-	$211,599	748	$1,126	$315	$282	$900	$1,395
V7283	OTH PREOP EXAM	$197,265	1,974	$567	$136	$99	$4,234	$575
78057	OTH SLEEP APNEA	$186,736	313	$2,288	$2,749	$596	$0	$1,960
2113	BEN NEO BOWEL	$180,566	369	$1,902	$527	$489	$5,859	$1,935
78650	CHEST PAIN NOS	$179,248	390	$2,380	$552	$459	$1,492	$2,014
5920	CALC OF KIDNEY	$174,352	104	$6,674	$1,732	$1,676	$1,692	$2,613
79439	ABN CARDIO STUD	$155,047	78	$7,568	$1,719	$1,987	$73	$5,820
V5332	Fit DFIBRILLATOR	$152,409	22	$34,412	$7,838	$6,927	$1,113	$16,407
20280	OTH LYMP UNSP	$139,535	112	$4,673	$1,224	$1,245	$7,146	$3,353
	All Other	$10,569,388	31,392	—	—	—	—	—
	TOTAL FOR ALL CLAIMS	$21,338,924	47,240	—	—	—	—	—

In table 4.7 one of the top five diagnoses is 285.9, Anemia NOS. This may raise a red flag for the level of precision in documentation. While only actual record review will confirm if a problem exists, this type of data review can justify investing in a record review. In table 4.8, the most expensive procedure is for a diagnostic cardiac catheterization (APC 0800). The charge alone for these cases may justify a review to validate that the documentation was accurate.

Documentation Review

Documentation review allows CDI professionals to verify whether problems seen in the data are being caused by clinical documentation that does not meet the criteria for high quality. Because they are reviewing only a sampling, they may need some additional verification. However, by using the suggestions that follow, the review should produce a result that is highly representative of the clinical documentation for the organization's overall patient base.

Table 4.8 Top 20 ambulatory payment classifications (APCs)

APC Number	APC Description	Total Payment	Number Patient Claims	Units of Service	Average Charge	Average Cost	Average Payment	National Average Charge
0300	Level I Rad Tx	$2,051,416	1,159	12,314	$541	$164	$166	$430
0080	Diag Card Cath	$959,830	501	501	$3,027	$738	$1,915	$3,688
0733	Non esrd epoetin alpha	$760,787	2,243	83,833	$95	$22	$9	$40
0304	Level I Rad TX	$618,749	3,296	7,200	$313	$95	$85	$317
0143	Lower GI Endo	$610,824	1,477	1,478	$1,275	$360	$413	$1,088
0612	High Lev ED Vis	$486,810	2,089	2,097	$634	$248	$232	$563
0303	TX Device Construction	$444,627	1,031	2,903	$524	$159	$153	$551
0260	Level I Xray	$425,613	8,816	10,192	$204	$39	$41	$171
0849	Rituximab, 100	$374,195	192	1,454	$1,954	$457	$257	$1,166
0206	Lev II Nerve Inj	$349,685	1,360	1,360	$630	$225	$257	$651
0714	New Tech Lev IX	$349,071	246	246	$4,016	$766	$1,418	$3,605
0332	CAT	$332,109	1,795	1,796	$1,042	$193	$184	$1,033
0280	Level III Angio	$318,244	429	451	$1,945	$494	$705	$1,623
0710	New Tech Lev V	$285,849	171	710	$2,726	$846	$402	$1,121
0823	Docetaxel,20 mg	$259,003	225	1,278	$1,249	$292	$202	$869
0267	Level III Dx Ultrasound	$254,713	1,921	1,926	$473	$185	$132	$561
0117	Chemo by Infus	$243,120	1,163	1,252	$602	$182	$194	$349
0905	Immune globulin	$234,727	265	8,281	$334	$78	$28	$172
0305	Level II TX Rad	$227,139	1,068	1,159	$770	$233	$195	$763
0291	Level II DX Nuc Med	$224,181	1,058	1,060	$820	$152	$211	$803
	TOT FOR TOP 20	$9,810,692	30,505	141,491	—	—	—	—
	SERV MIX IND =	2.575						

www.ahd.com. Used with permission.

Concurrent Versus Retrospective Review

There are two ways to review clinical documentation in patient records—concurrently or retrospectively. Reviewing records concurrently requires the reviewer to be on the unit where the patient is being treated. The concurrent review takes place after documentation has been recorded, but before the patient has been discharged. While technically, this is not a concurrent review of the documentation, it is a review concurrent with the patient's stay.

In a retrospective review, the documentation is assessed after the patient has been discharged and usually after the record has been coded. The retrospective review can take place prior to billing or after billing depending on the organization's common policies and procedures. The advantage to reviewing records after coding, but prior to billing, is that if there are changes made that would affect the coding, they can be made before the bill is submitted. The disadvantage to reviewing records prior to billing is that it significantly limits the population from which the sample is drawn, thereby possibly making the findings less reliable. Table 4.9 lists the advantages and disadvantages of both the concurrent and the retrospective approaches to record review. Another option to consider is performing a review that includes both a retrospective and a current review.

Table 4.9   Advantages and disadvantages of concurrent and retrospective reviews

Review Type	Advantages	Disadvantages
Concurrent	• Real time intervention with physicians to make changes identified during the audit • Greater reliability of the recommended query • Ability to mimic the activity of a clinical documentation program and provide subjective information about how successful the actual process could be	• Review time and cost can be increased significantly because the reviewers must locate cases unit by unit • Sample selection is not random, so the findings will not be generalizable to the entire patient population
Retrospective	• Review time and cost is less than concurrent review since records can be identified and pulled prior to starting the work • Random sample selection is possible, making the results of the review generalizable across the entire patient population	• The ability to determine a concurrent query retrospectively may be difficult in some cases and may result in under or over estimation of the impact • The ability to act on any findings that may impact reimbursement may be limited due to payer time constraints

Collecting a Sample for Retrospective Review

Some of the initial issues to consider for sampling include identifying the population, determining the size of the sample, and selecting the methodology to be used. Identifying and documenting the population is an important first step (Babbie 1999). For example, some organizations may exclude normal newborn cases or certain one-day stay cases from their documentation review. When any segment of the population is excluded, the exclusion as well as the rationale for eliminating these cases should be documented. Recording the information allows for replication of the study for future comparisons.

Once the population has been clarified, the sample size must be determined. A documentation review needs to be representative, but not necessarily scientific. Any sample must contain at least 30 cases to be reliable (Babbie 1999; Alreck and Settle 1995). Ideally, the sample should be based on the number of discharges and, for at least a 90 percent confidence interval, a sample size of between 100 and 200 is likely to represent a good number for any organization (Wang et al. 1995, 53). Some organizations may engage statisticians and apply other methodologies for sample selection. The most important consideration is that, over time, the organization will want to use the same methodology for all sample selections. This will allow the results to be comparable. If the methodology is modified, even slightly, results will not be comparable from study to study.

After determining the number of cases in the sample, the methodology to select the records must be determined. Random sampling is optimal since it will be generally representative of the overall patient population (Babbie 1999), and a representative sample is most likely to yield study findings that a CDI review team would be likely to identify as opportunities for improvement. Some organizations stratify by payer or even service. But ultimately, if the sample size is large enough, it will include cases that are representative of the entire patient population.

Collecting a Sample for Concurrent Review

Unless the organization is fairly large with several hundred discharges per day, it will be impossible to obtain a random sample selection for an efficient concurrent review. One way to approach the concurrent review process is to replicate the activities of a CDI program. Essentially, reviewers conduct their assessment of the records in the same manner that clinical documentation specialists would. While an organization cannot generalize the results of such a review over the entire patient population, it can report on the findings as representative of a two-week period of CDI review. If a review is approached in this manner, it is best to couple it with a retrospective review of at least 100 records.

There is a way to conduct a concurrent review using a random-type sampling methodology (Babbie 1999). It will not be as reliable as the sample selection methodology for retrospective review, but it can provide more representative results than the scenario previously described. First, the reviewers must be prepared to spread out the review over a four- to eight-week period so that sampling is not biased by the short timeframe. Smaller hospitals should use the eight-week time period, while larger hospitals can use the four-week time period. Each day, using the census listing, a random number of patients is selected for review. If the patient was already reviewed, that patient's record is thrown out and a replacement record is added. By using random number generators found on the Internet, this sample selection will be as objective as possible.

Reviewing the Documentation

When reviewing records for clinical documentation, it is most important to focus the review solely on the documentation. When the review is retrospective, the reviewer may have a tendency to be influenced by the coding assigned to the records. Thus, reviewing the records without referencing the coding would provide the most reliable results.

The review should be performed by individuals with clinical expertise as well as training in clinical documentation review. In organizations that do not have clinical documentation experts available internally, a team of a nurse reviewer and a coding professional can provide the appropriate skill set. The team, however, must be trained in the principles of high-quality clinical documentation as well as the organization's specific objectives for the review. The objectives become very important during the analysis phase. In this phase, the review team should identify not only opportunities for querying physicians, but also what the impact would be if the response was positive. For example, in some cases, a query response may change the coding, the DRG assignment, or both. In other cases, the query response may change reporting for quality indicators. In other cases, the response may impact severity leveling, while in others it may impact more than one performance outcome.

The most reliable and consistent methodology for reviewing clinical documentation is to use the criteria for high-quality clinical documentation to identify wherever documentation is deficient (Russo 2008). This methodology will also ensure that the review is compliant. When a query is recommended, especially in a retrospective review, it is best to have the agreement of at least two reviewers before including it in a final report.

Reporting and Acting on Findings

The primary purpose of the report of findings from the clinical documentation review is to determine whether the review has identified one or more problems with the quality of clinical documentation. If the answer is yes, then additional detail should be added to the report to specify the number and type of problems found. Of most importance is to state the findings in an objective, factual format. Then, the report can be used to draw logical conclusions based on the data. Some examples of how to report the findings are discussed. The report should include detailed data specific to the needs and goals of the organization. Table 4.10 shows the differences in severity levels if the documentation in the records reviewed was complete on the units or at the time of coding. In the best case scenario, if documentation was completed concurrently, the percentage of level 3 cases would increase from 22 percent to 32 percent. This finding alone could support the recommendation to implement a complete CDI program.

Table 4.11 is an example of a CMI analysis performed on the records in the review. The current CMI is listed along with projected CMI. Projected CMI is CMI with improved clinical documentation. The actual CMI opportunity can be calculated by adding up all of the relative weight differences from the review and dividing that number by the total number of discharges for the payer for a year. In table 4.11, the overall Medicare impact would be about .063. The economic value of that opportunity is determined by multiplying the improved opportunity (.063) by the hospital's blended rate.

The conclusion to the clinical documentation review process is a decision to move forward (or not) with a CDI program. The more careful thought and preparation that goes into the assessment process, the more reliable and sustainable the CDI program that emanates from it is likely to be.

Conclusion

A clinical documentation assessment is an important prerequisite to a implementing a CDI program. First, the organization's data should be reviewed for inconsistencies and/or patterns that do not meet target norms. Second, using results of the data review, clinical documentation in patient records should be assessed. The sample and the methodology for review should be carefully selected, and the same methods used for each review so results can be compared over time. Finally, results should be gathered, findings analyzed, recommendations made, and the report prepared and delivered to the appropriate managers in the organization.

Table 4.10   Differences in severity levels depending on documentation

Severity Level	Current Documentation	Complete Documentation at Coding	Complete Concurrent Documentation
Minor (Level 1)	20%	17%	15%
Moderate (Level 2)	57%	54%	51%
Major (Level 3)	22%	28%	32%
Extreme (Level 4)	1%	1%	2%

Table 4.11   Case mix index (CMI) comparison analysis

Medicare Payers only:			
	Current	Projected	Opportunity
Medical CMI:	1.0635	1.1107	+ .0472
Surgical CMI:	2.4615	2.4781	+ .0166
All Other Payers:			
	Current	Projected	Opportunity
Medical CMI:	0.8033	0.8424	+ .0391
Surgical CMI:	1.8921	1.9249	+ .0328

References

Alreck, P. L., and R. B. Settle. 1995. *The Survey Research Handbook.* New York City: McGraw Hill.

American Hospital Directory (AHD). 2008. http://www.ahd.com/.

Babbie, E. 1999. *The Basics of Social Research.* Albany, NY: Wadsworth Publishing Company.

Centers for Medicare and Medicaid Services. 2008. *Public Quality Indicator and Resident Reports.* http://www.cms.hhs.gov/MDSPubQIandResRep/.

Drucker, P. 1999. Knowledge worker productivity: The biggest challenge. *California Management Review* 41(2):83–94.

IPRO. 2005a. Coding for Quality: Documentation Tips for the Top Seven DRGs Revised 2005, Hospital Payment Monitoring Program. http://providers.ipro.org/index/hpmp.

IPRO. 2005b. Coding for Quality: Documentation tips for the Top Ten Denied DRGs, Hospital Payment Monitoring Program. http://providers.ipro.org/index/hpmp.

Pennsylvania Health Care Cost Containment Council (PHCCC). 2006. *Cardiac Surgery in Pennsylvania 2005–2006.* http://www.phc4.org/reports/cabg/06/docs/cabg2006keyfindings.pdf.

Russo, R. 2008. *A Compelling Case for Clinical Documentation.* Bethlehem, PA: DJ Iber Publishing.

Wang, M. Q., E. Fitzhugh, and R. C. Westerfield. 1995. Determining sample sizes for simple random surveys. *Health Values* 19(3):53–56.

Chapter 5
Moving Forward

Making the decision to move forward with a clinical documentation improvement (CDI) program is an essential choice for every organization. The decision should be based on an objective assessment of the organization's current clinical documentation practices. Using this information, the organization should create a vision statement for its CDI program, and include the goals for the CDI staff (Russo 2008). In addition, the organization must be prepared to support the program with appropriate resources and staffing. This chapter addresses the crafting of a vision statement for CDI and how to gain the necessary organizational support for the program.

Key Decision Makers

Before proceeding with the creation of a vision statement for clinical documentation and the CDI program, it is necessary to have the right individuals in place to participate in the decision-making process. The CDI leadership has one chance to make a good decision that will be embraced by the organization. Leaving out a key player during the visioning process can mean failure, or at the very least, a significant setback for the program.

Because CDI is an interdisciplinary process, it is essential to include leaders in each of the functional areas that impact the CDI process. While each organization will vary, in general, suggested participants include:

- Chief medical officer (CMO)

- Chief financial officer (CFO)

- Other key physicians, especially from areas that show high opportunity

- Director of health information management

- Director of case management

- Chief compliance officer

- Director of quality

- Chief information officer (CIO) (or appropriate representative from information technology)

- Emergency medical room (EMR) project leader (if an EMR is implemented or is being implemented)

- Chief nursing officer (depending on the organization)

- Vice president of outpatient services (if outpatient services are in the scope of the client need)

Creating a Vision for Clinical Documentation and the Clinical Documentation Improvement Program

When developing a new CDI program or improving an existing one within the organization, CDI leadership needs to ask the following question before spending any (or any more) of the organization's resources on this effort. Why do we want to improve clinical documentation? The essence of the question is: What does our organization hope to achieve by implementing a new or upgrading a current CDI program?

In developing a CDI vision statement, the organization should begin with its own values, vision, and mission statements. The CDI vision statement should flow naturally from these broader statements about what the healthcare organization values, and where it is going. The CDI vision statement does two things. First, it provides a purpose for the program. Second, it provides a way to get the attention of the physicians and other clinicians whose documentation the effort is attempting to improve.

Research shows that unless the vision is specific to the program and the organization, it is unlikely to succeed and be sustained (Porras and Collins 1996; Collins 2001). Some of the reasons for implementing a CDI program include the following:

- The healthcare team caring for the patient has an interest in the highest-quality clinical documentation. Without complete and accurate documentation, the best treatment is not possible. The healthcare team provides one of the strongest arguments for having a CDI program: high-quality care for patients.

- Organizations that measure quality use the hospital's publicly available data to create quality scorecards for the hospital. These scorecards rate the hospital by type of diagnosis treated and surgical procedures performed (http://www.healthgrades.com/), how the hospital treated certain diagnoses (Medicare quality indicators [http://www.cms.hhs.gov/] and the Leapfrog Group [http://www.leapfroggroup.org/]), and how frequently certain surgeries were performed (https://www.vimo.com/) among others. The organization's *perceived quality,* which is the public's perception of its quality care based on these reports, is driven by the clinical documentation in the patient records.

- Patients have a greater interest in obtaining, maintaining, and understanding their patient records. The patient owns the information in the record and, under HIPAA, the patient has the right to ask someone in the organization to explain the content, correct it, or even rewrite the information if it is illegible (HIPAA 1996). The motivation for high-quality clinical documentation in this instance is patient satisfaction. Requests by patients to review their records have increased in recent years. Well-kept, easy-to-read, complete health records will likely begin to play a more prominent role in patient satisfaction (Gunter 2002).

- An organization's healthcare planning relies, to a large extent, on the data it gathers (Johnson 2001). Organizations use details about types of patients being treated, how patients are being treated, and clinical details about symptoms and diagnoses. All this information is generated from the clinical documentation in health records that is translated into coded data by health information management professionals. The organization needs accurate and complete information to make good decisions (Russo 2008).

- The same clinical documentation is also used in medical malpractice or other legal claims against the hospital, as the basis for payment by health plans, and for research and reporting to government and regulatory agencies. These examples are more operational in nature than the first four uses mentioned.

Healthcare organizations should consider all of these issues when creating a CDI vision statement. Ultimately, a CDI vision statement should embrace the issues that CDI leadership believes are most significant to the organization and be a natural extension of the organization's overall mission statement.

Initial Structure: Program Committees

This section presents CDI structures that have proven to be effective in over 100 CDI programs where the author personally assisted in implementing or redesigning the program. The initial structure for a CDI program, in most organizations, should be two guided committees. Smaller organizations may only need one committee or ad hoc group, but most will need a committee that operates at the strategic level of the organization and another that operates at the day-to-day, or operational, level of the organization. Over time, these committees may change into a formalized department with an executive team member who is responsible for clinical documentation and CDI practices. Most organizations should begin with the committee structure and determine, over time, what long-term structure will work best in their environment to support and maintain high-quality clinical documentation.

Oversight Committee

Support from the top is essential to the success of a CDI program. Therefore, the oversight committee should be composed of members of executive management, the physician advisor or leader for clinical documentation and CDI, and the manager of the CDI program. In general, the oversight committee should include the CEO, CFO, CMO, chief compliance officer, CIO, a physician, CDI leader, and CDI program manager. Committee composition may vary by the size and complexity of the organization. For example in a very large organization, the vice president of operations or the COO may sit on the committee in lieu of the CEO, and a vice president of reimbursement may sit on the committee in lieu of the CFO.

The amount of time that the committee needs to spend in meetings gradually decreases for the initial kick-off of the program, it is best for all members of both the oversight and the day-to-day committees to meet. At this meeting, specific responsibilities of each group are reviewed. The chair of the oversight committee manages this meeting with the chair of the operations committee. During this joint committee meeting, each group agrees to its responsibilities and communicates its expectations about what is needed from the other group. During the initial implementation phase, the oversight committee may meet every other week. Then, during the remainder of the first year, the oversight committee should meet monthly. During year two, when additions and adjustments are being made to the program, the oversight committee may meet every quarter. Finally, as clinical documentation and CDI becomes an operationalized function within the organization, the oversight committee will likely stop meeting. The responsibilities of the oversight committee however, do not stop. They are usually overtaken by a standing executive-level committee, often a quality initiative or other strategic committee.

During its time of operation, the oversight committee has five key responsibilities. First, the group must obtain and maintain support from the medical staff. This is the most essential role that the oversight committee plays. Initially, the committee must determine the strategy for obtaining physician support and, through its own actions, demonstrate the importance of the CDI initiative. In addition to obtaining support, the oversight committee should also determine the chain of command that will be used to manage physicians who are either unresponsive or uncooperative with the CDI program staff. The oversight committee is responsible for obtaining initial program funding through the organization's budget and maintaining that funding for some period, usually up to two years. After that time, the function has likely been operationalized and is included as a budget line item. The oversight committee should also identify the key metrics it will use to measure program success. This committee reviews those metrics regularly and provides feedback to the operations group on how they perceive the program is moving. Table 5.1 summarizes the responsibilities of the oversight committee.

Operational Committee

The operational committee is made up of the individuals who are responsible for the day-to-day management of and support for the CDI program. The members of this committee are likely to include the CDI program manager, physician leader for CDI, health information manager, coding manager, quality indicators manager, data analyst, financial analyst, or case mix manager. Depending on the structure of the program, the director of case management may also participate on this committee. The quality indicators manager is the individual in the organization who supervises the abstraction of data for quality indicators purposes. Because of the overlap in responsibilities, someone from this function should be involved in CDI so that any synergies that would allow the organization to operate more efficiently can be identified and implemented. A data analyst (or similar individual) should be involved so that data can be easily accessed. CDI specialists may or may not be involved with the committee. Generally, for organizations with a large number of CDI specialists (five or more), they will not be included in the operations meetings. But, for organizations with only a few CDI specialists, they may be included in the meetings. In smaller organizations, the CDI specialists are likely to play a role in program management and may be multitasking within the program. In this case, it may make sense to include all members in the operations committee. For larger organizations, including all CDI specialists would be inefficient for program operations. Because of the operational nature of the CDI program, a member of the compliance team should not be included in this group. The day-to-day operational involvement of a compliance team member could conflict with the CDI specialist's responsibilities for reviewing and auditing organizational activities.

Table 5.1   Clinical documentation oversight committee responsibilities

Oversight committee responsibilities
•   Obtain and maintain medical staff support
•   Create a *chain of command* to manage uncooperative physicians
•   Support the program financially
•   Determine key metrics to be reviewed at the strategic level
•   Provide feedback to the CDI operational group

The operations committee should meet weekly during the first few months of the program. There are a significant number of activities that need to be coordinated, and the weekly meetings will help facilitate these. After the first few months, the operations committee will meet monthly for the first two years of program operation. In the second year, members of the committee may be changed. For example, the data analyst and financial analyst may no longer be needed on the committee.

There are seven primary responsibilities of the operations committee. They include the initial responsibilities of hiring and training program staff as well as training physicians and other clinicians in high-quality clinical documentation practices. As the CDI program staff members are hired and trained, they will assume more and more of the operational responsibilities. And, the operational committee will play a support and review function. On an ongoing basis, the operations committee is responsible for ensuring the query process along with any other activities necessary to obtain high-quality clinical documentation. Other responsibilities of the operations committee include reviewing CDI program data, supervising the design of auditing clinical documentation and CDI functions, supervising the design of follow-up training for physicians, and reporting on key metrics to the oversight committee. The responsibilities of the operations committee are included in table 5.2.

One caveat should be noted for organizations that are small and focused. In organizations with fewer than 50 beds, the committee structure will be greatly streamlined, and individuals may take on the roles of multiple members of a committee. The committee structures recommended above assume that an organization is operating with at least 150 beds. Organizations with fewer than 150 inpatient beds should use the suggested committee structures to determine which activities need to be performed and then assign individuals to those roles. The activities that need to be completed remain the same regardless of the size of the organization. Each organization will just need to determine how it can best accomplish those activities.

Figure 5.1 demonstrates a typical committee structure for a clinical documentation program.

Communicating to the Organization

As with any new function, it is necessary for an organization to undertake a strategic communications process about clinical documentation and the CDI program to ensure the success and sustainability of the program. This is really part of the oversight committee's responsibility for obtaining support from the medical staff for the CDI program. The operations committee is involved in disseminating the message, but the initial

Table 5.2   Clinical documentation operations committee responsibilities

Operations committee responsibilities
• Hire and train staff
• Oversee the training of physicians and other clinicians
• Implement and oversee activities to obtain high-quality clinical documentation through day-to-day activities such as querying, record review, and one-on-one training with physicians
• Review program data for tracking and measuring
• Supervise the design of auditing clinical documentation and clinical documentation improvement functions
• Supervise the design of follow-up training for physicians
• Report on key metrics to the oversight committee

Figure 5.1   Clinical documentation committee structure

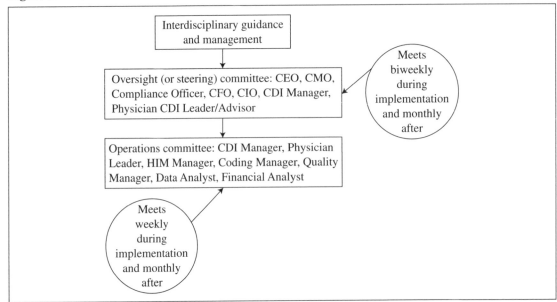

communication must come from the top of the organization. The message about clinical documentation and the CDI program that comes from the CEO and other executives in the organization is evidence to the physicians of the importance of both the program and the physicians' participation in the program.

The Communication Process

Communication about the CDI process should begin in advance of any training or operationalizing of the program. Letting the physicians know about the program is a way to prepare them for the coming activities and, if done appropriately, it can also be used to obtain the physicians' support for the program. The organization should consider three key concepts. First, who will the communication come from? Second, what media should be used to communicate? And third, what information will be communicated? The initial communication about the program should come from the CEO of the organization. It is important to start at the top, so the CEO should be involved. Subsequent communications can come from the CMO or the physician leader for CDI. The media that is selected to communicate may vary since physicians in each organization may value one type of communication over another. The primary means of communication include in-person meetings, letters, and e-mail. The best way to communicate is through multiple media. For example, an in-person meeting with the CEO and members of the medical staff, in which the CEO discusses the program and then follows up with an e-mail or hard copy letter (depending on the organization), is likely to send the most powerful message (Patterson et al. 2002).

Once the message has been communicated to physicians and all managers in the organization about the program, follow up with additional communications is needed. These communications should come from a physician. The importance of physician involvement is discussed later in this section. These communications should begin to introduce the physicians to more details about the CDI program and the CDI program staff. Some details about the staff's qualifications, the training programs, and query process should be shared in these communications. If e-mail is used, each e-mail should be dedicated to one aspect of the program since most physicians are not likely to read the contents of a lengthy e-mail.

Some organizations have successfully used marketing communications in addition to personal communications to announce the CDI program. For example, organizations have used posters in the physicians' lounge and announcements and brief articles in the medical staff newsletter. These tactics may be helpful in some organizations, but they should only be used after a formal communication is sent from the CEO and CMO to the medical staff. Members of the medical staff should not find out about a CDI program initially by reading a brochure or poster in the lounge. Marketing materials should supplement the personal message and not be used as the initial means of communication. Figure 5.2 shows a sample letter to the medical staff from the CEO describing the CDI program.

Once it has been determined who will communicate the information and how it will be communicated, it is essential to determine the exact message. The beginning of this chapter addressed the importance of creating a program vision that is linked directly to the organization's vision and mission statements. The concepts of quality of care, perceived quality, and patient satisfaction were identified as key reasons for implementation of a program. These reasons are important to physicians and should be included in the message. While accurate reimbursement is usually a key goal of a CDI program, it should not be the only goal and should not be communicated to the medical staff as the primary reason for the program.

Physicians should understand how the goals of the CDI program align with their goals. If an organization has identified quality and patient satisfaction goals as the vision for CDI, these goals will probably strike a chord with the physicians. It is important to include this information in the initial message to them. In addition, there are benefits to the physicians that result when they improve their clinical documentation in the hospital. This should be part of the communication as well. Next, the message should communicate what the hospital's expectations are regarding physicians' involvement in the CDI process. The physicians' responsibilities should be explained realistically, but with a focus on using a limited amount of their time. Finally, the message should share with the physicians any benefits they can expect from the hospital. This may include a meal during the training program and CME credits. The sample letter in figure 5.2 summarizes the information to be communicated to physicians.

Physicians

Physician support is the key to the success and sustainability of the CDI program. The organization should identify initial physician supporters prior to the formal communications about the program. In addition to the CMO or vice president of medical affairs, the program should have a physician advisor or leader CDI by the time the announcement has been made. The physician leader's name can be included on communications so other physicians can contact the leader with questions about the program. In addition, the organization should create a strategy that brings other physician leaders into the fold to support CDI as early as possible. Who exactly is pulled in will vary by organization.

The chiefs of service may be a good group to involve. If the organization employs physicians (hospitalists, physician group practices, or others) they should all learn about the program prior to the initial communication to the medical staff. These individuals can help clarify questions other physicians may have. They can also demonstrate support for the process. Other physicians that an organization may want to inform early in the process include the *informal* medical staff leaders. These are the physicians who everyone respects and goes to with problems, but they do not hold a specific position within the organization. Every organization has a few of these leaders. It may be wise for the CMO or the CEO to meet with these physicians individually prior to the initial announcement. An informal lunch where CDI is discussed along with other key initiatives of the organization, can solidify support from these informal leaders. The more physician support the organization obtains for the CDI program in its early stages, the higher the likelihood of success and sustainability.

Figure 5.2   Sample letter from the CEO to the medical staff

Date

James Smith, MD
214 Elm Street
Providence, RI 10034

Re: Clinical Documentation Program

I hope you were able to attend the medical staff meeting last week where I described the hospital's clinical documentation program, which will begin in March. I wanted to provide you with some additional detail about the program. As well as the benefits to our organization overall, the program will provide you with some documentation training opportunities that you can use in your private practice as well as with patients in the hospital.

Research has shown that physician clinical documentation in patient records is directly linked to quality indicators, quality of care, and the efficiency of healthcare operations. In addition, patients are twice as likely to request and read copies of their health records today than they were 10 years ago. And, under HIPAA patients have the right to request modifications to their health information. Based upon this research and our desire to maintain high quality care and high levels of patient satisfaction, we are implementing a clinical documentation program. This program teaches the criteria for high quality clinical documentation and program staff use the criteria to review patient records for opportunities for improvement.

I am asking for your support of this clinical documentation initiative. Your responsibilities to the program include attendance at an initial documentation training program and continued attendance at follow-up training two to three times per year. In return, the hospital will provide you with lunch or dinner and CMEs for every hour of training you attend. In addition, you may be asked to clarify documentation in your patient records by one of the clinical documentation specialists, who will be located on the nursing units. If asked, you will need to clarify your documentation in the patient's record.

If you have any questions about the program or would like additional information on the research conducted to justify implementing the program, I would be happy to share that with you. You can also find additional information about the program, including program staff names and contact information, in the physicians' lounge and in the current medical staff newsletter.

Thank you for your time and involvement in this process. I appreciate the work you do with our healthcare system and the contributions that your practice of medicine makes to our community.

Sincerely,

CEO

cc:

CFO, CMO, CIO, Compliance Officer (Oversight Committee Members)

Conclusion

It is essential for every organization to develop a vision statement for its CDI program. This statement will guide the organization and its physicians towards the ultimate key outcomes of CDI: high-quality care, high perceived quality, improved patient satisfaction, and accurate reimbursement. It is important to involve the right individuals when creating the vision. It is also important to involve physicians in the vision process as well as in the initial communication process to the medical staff. The CEO should take the lead in communicating with the medical staff about the CDI program. However, physician leaders and physician employees throughout the organization should be informed about the program first so they can be available to respond to questions and concerns that members of the medical staff may have about the CDI program. These activities are likely to improve the success and sustainability of the program.

References

Collins, J. 2001. *Good to Great: Why Some Companies Make the Leap and Others Don't.* New York: Harper Collins Publishers.

Gunter, K. 2002. The HIPAA privacy rule: Practical advice for academic and research institutions. *Healthcare Financial Management.* 56(2):50–56.

HIPAA Privacy Rule. 1996. 45 CFR Part 160 and Subparts A and E of Part 164; http://www.access.gpo.gov/nara/cfr/waisidx_07/45cfr160_07.html.

Johnson, D. E. 2001. HIPAA is a new weapon and career opportunity. *Heath Care Strategic Management.* 19(2):2–3.

Patterson, K., J. Grenny, R. McMillan, A. Switzler. 2002. *Crucial Conversations: Tools for Talking When Stakes are High.* New York: McGraw Hill.

Porras, G., and J. Collins. 1996. *Built to Last: Successful Habits of Visionary Companies.* New York: Harper Collins Publishers.

Russo, R. 2008. *A Compelling Case for Clinical Documentation: Use Clinical Documentation to Achieve Strategic Alignment with Your Medical Staff.* (Volume 1). Bethlehem, PA: DJ Iber Publishing.

Russo, R. 2008. *A Compelling Case for Clinical Documentation: Use the CAMP Method to Improve Clinical Documentation Quality.* (Volume 2) Bethlehem, PA: DJ Iber Publishing.

Part 2
Implementing a Clinical Documentation Program

Chapter 6
Staffing the Program

The clinical documentation improvement (CDI) program needs a structure to ensure continued success and sustainability. When considering the structure to support the program, an organization must address clinical documentation at four levels: reporting, management, staffing, and physician leadership. General guidelines for staffing and management should be applied within the context of the dynamics of the organization. Every organization is unique in its culture and dynamics. Ultimate success in clinical documentation depends on tailoring the program's structure to fit the organization.

Program Reporting

Before making any structural determinations, an organization should decide to whom the CDI program will ultimately report. Because the program involves clinical documentation and relies upon the physicians for success, the CMO or vice president of the medical staff is the optimal reporting structure. In organizations with a new or less than optimal medical staff management function, it may be necessary to design a different short-term strategy. Implementation of a new function requires strong leadership. The recommendations presented in this chapter can be used to develop the best long-term strategy for management and support of the CDI program, but in the short term, the CDI program may need to report into another administrative function that ultimately reports to the CEO or COO, with a dotted-line reporting relationship to the CMO.

Physician Leaders

Physician leadership is essential to a successful and sustainable CDI program (Marco and Buchman 2003; Keogh and Martin 2004). Ideally, a program should incorporate four levels of physician leadership: two official levels and two unofficial levels. The two official levels of leadership include the physician at the executive level and the physician who is designated as the CDI program advisor or leader. In addition, the organization should develop physician CDI leaders within the medical staff and within the physician management team.

First, the physician executive in charge of the CDI program should preferably be the CMO or the vice president of medical affairs. This executive must be involved with the design and communications of the clinical documentation program from the start. The physician executive should also be involved in identifying other physicians who support and manage the program and who encourage the entire medical staff.

Second, the CDI program must have a physician who is officially designated as the physician leader for CDI. Ideally, this physician should be a full-time employee of the hospital. But, for smaller organizations, the physician may be a part-time employee. Organizations without appropriate resources to support the program with physician management, can contract with an external organization that has expertise in clinical documentation. This strategy should be a temporary one until the organization can secure its own physician leader for the program.

The physician leader for CDI should have experience and expertise consistent with the responsibilities demanded by the CDI program, as listed in table 6.1. The physician leader must be involved in all formal training provided to physicians. The physician leader also serves in a support role to the CDI program specialists. The leader should be available to answer questions the program staff may have and assist in particularly challenging reviews. When the CDI specialist encounters a problematic physician, the physician leader should be responsible for obtaining cooperation from the physician. The physician leader for CDI should serve on the oversight and operations committees. Finally, the physician leader should oversee the clinical documentation audits and be prepared to make judgment calls when there are particularly challenging documentation problems. Ideally, the physician CDI program leader should report directly to the CMO. Depending on the size of the organization and whether the physician leader for CDI is a full-time employee, the physician may manage the entire CDI function, or the function may report directly to the CMO or other executive level manager. Table 6.1 presents the general responsibilities of the physician leader for CDI.

The physician leader for CDI should have certain experience and qualifications. Ideally, the physician leader should be well-versed in the principles of high quality clinical documentation, but this is a skill that can be learned if the right individual can be identified to do the job. Other characteristics and experience that the physician leader should have include:

- The ability to negotiate well with peers
- Recent or current active medical practice
- Record review and teaching experience

Table 6.1   Responsibilities of the physician leader for CDI

Responsibilities of the Physician Leader for CDI
• Conducts initial and follow-up clinical documentation training with program staff
• Manages physician responsiveness to queries and cooperation with program staff
• Supports CDI specialists
• Assists in CDI reviews that are particularly challenging
• Manages clinical documentation audits
• Serves on the oversight and operations CDI committees

Table 6.2   Qualifications of a physician leader for CDI

Skill	Ideal	Minimum
Formal education	Currently licensed MD or DO; board certified in specialty of physicians in the training group	Currently licensed MD or DO
Training received in clinical documentation	40 hours or more, certification	At least 40 hours
Experience in Clinical Documentation	5 years of practice; currently treating patients	3 years of practice and currently treating patients on at least a part-time basis
Experience providing classroom instruction	40 hours or more of classroom instruction	At least 40 hours of classroom instruction
Experience providing practical instruction	100 hours or more of on-unit or in-office instruction including observation and feedback	At least 40 hours of on-unit or in-office instruction including observation and feedback
Communication	Ability to negotiate with peers	Ability to negotiate with peers

When the physician identified as the physician leader for CDI does not have existing expertise in CDI, the organization can bring in an external physician to teach and temporarily supplement the responsibilities of the physician leader (Russo 2008). Table 6.2 contains the qualifications of a physician leader for CDI. The table includes two columns, one for the ideal qualifications and one for minimum qualifications. Because it is so difficult to find physicians who are trained in the CDI process, organizations can use the minimum qualifications to identify a physician who can then be trained on CDI processes.

In addition to the official physician program support, it is also important to ensure that the structure allows for the development of unofficial physician supporters for the CDI program. This activity should be a designated responsibility of both the CMO (regardless of the reporting relationship) and the physician leader for CDI. These leaders should be charged with obtaining support for CDI from service chiefs, any physicians employed by the healthcare organization, and the unofficial physician leaders who are on the medical staff. The CMO is likely to have more success with obtaining support from physicians in most of these situations, but the physician leader for CDI should be involved in the relationship development activities as well.

Program Management

The structure of the program will depend on the size of the organization as well as how many functions within the organization will be staffed initially for CDI. Ideally, the program should be directed by a full-time CDI manager who reports to the CMO. However, except in large organizations or organizations with long-term CDI in all areas, this structure is unlikely to be either effective or efficient for the organization. It is probable that the CDI program manager will report into a director for another function, at least initially. Therefore, both program management and the day-to-day department reporting structure should be addressed in the CDI program structure.

If clinical documentation will not be an independent department initially in the organization, where does it belong? Common, workable options include the departments of health information management, case management, and quality management. The specific criteria for choosing a department that will house the CDI function include the following:

- The efficiency and effectiveness of the department in the past—The best choice is a department that has met or exceeded its key metrics consistently for at least the last three to five years. It is difficult for an efficiently run department to take on a new responsibility and nearly impossible for an inefficient department to do so.

- A visionary department director—CDI is a new concept for most organizations. The manager of the CDI function must be capable of creative, out-of-the-box thinking for the program to be successful. A well-oiled department with a manager who has been responsible for the same three functions for the past 10 years is probably not the best choice for housing the CDI function.

Every organization is different in terms of strengths and weaknesses. If these criteria are applied in choosing where the function will be located, chances of success are increased (Grol et al. 2002).

Except in very small organizations, the CDI program needs its own manager. This individual is responsible for managing the clinical documentation staff, all training and the query process, collecting program data, and reporting key metrics, as well as representing the CDI program as a committee member. In some organizations, the CDI program manager may also be responsible for reviewing records on the unit and querying physicians when appropriate. The CDI program manager interacts regularly with the physician leader for CDI.

The CDI program manager should have some clinical background, record review experience, and extensive training experience, especially with physicians. In addition, the manager should have experience with healthcare coding and reimbursement systems. The manager must also be able to communicate effectively with physicians, to motivate staff, and be comfortable with ambiguity and change. Since the CDI program is a new function in the organization and will need to morph to become a functional operations unit some day, the CDI manager must be able to look ahead. Figure 6.1 shows a sample position description for a CDI program manager. This organization combined the CDI manager position duties with some reimbursement-related activities to make the position into a full-time position. Depending on the needs of an organization, the specifics of the duties for the CDI manager may vary.

Program Staff

The CDI program staff members, or CDI specialists, are responsible for the day-to-day activities of the program. Initially, the primary activities are training and record review. Once initial training has been provided to all physicians and clinicians, the program staff focus on record review, querying, and ongoing physician education. They may also be involved in conducting follow-up education with physicians. In addition, as clinical documentation activities are expanded into various patient care areas, the CDI specialists may have the opportunity to take on additional responsibilities.

Figure 6.1   Clinical documentation improvement manager position description

---

Job Description: Clinical Documentation Improvement Manager

General description:
The manager of documentation improvement and reimbursement is responsible for ensuring that clinical documentation within the health system is consistent with the services and care provided to patients. The manager acts as a coordinator of physician clinical documentation, coding, and reimbursement processes in working towards high-quality clinical documentation and meeting key metrics for all services provided in the system.

Experience:

The successful candidate should:

1. Have a minimum of five years work experience in coding and health information management with progressive management responsibilities
2. Be familiar with all government healthcare reimbursement systems
3. Have experience working collaboratively with diverse groups in a healthcare environment
4. Be successful in interacting effectively with physicians
5. Possess excellent speaking, writing, and teaching skills
6. Have the ability to analyze large amounts of data to identify trends

Education:

1. Bachelor's degree in health information management, nursing, or equivalent
2. Current certification in a health information management or coding discipline recommended
3. If not a clinician, must have completed clinical coursework with the ability to understand disease processes

Specific responsibilities:
Interdisciplinary:
The manager of documentation improvement and reimbursement will function primarily as an interdisciplinary functional manager who focuses on ensuring physician documentation meets criteria for high quality clinical documentation. To that end, the manager will have access to physicians and clinical staff to participate in and assist in ensuring the ongoing documentation improvement effort is successful.

The manager:

1. Coordinates the activities of the documentation improvement committee
2. Ensures that the documentation improvement committee is continuously used primarily as a vehicle to promote documentation improvement for accurate reimbursement on an ongoing basis
3. Oversees the documentation improvement efforts of clinical documentation specialists and other program staff as necessary
4. Provides ongoing education to medical staff on documentation concerns
5. Works with finance department on continuous case mix modeling and assessment
6. Participates in the rejections and claims review process with patient accounting to ensure both compliance and accurate reimbursement
7. Tracks trends in documentation concerns and implementing corrective action
8. Directs coding activities to ensure accurate, consistent, and compliant coding for all services
9. Creates and updates documentation tools on an ongoing basis
10. Uses the claims denials, auditing, and testing processes to design and conduct follow-up CDI education with physicians

---

(continued on next page)

Figure 6.1   Clinical documentation improvement manager position description *(continued)*

Inpatient services:
1. Tracks case mix through both retrospective and concurrent means

2. Provides feedback to clinical documentation improvement specialists, case managers, coders, physicians, and other clinicians involved in the documentation improvement effort

3. Recommends and implements corrective actions when deficiencies are identified

Outpatient services:
1. Designs a case mix tracking system for APCs

2. Implements a documentation improvement program for outpatient services

3. Recommends and implements corrective actions when deficiencies are identified

Physician services:
1. Designs a documentation proficiency tracking system for system-based pro-fee billing and coding

2. Implements a documentation improvement program for pro-fee billing and coding

3. Recommends and implements corrective actions when deficiencies are identified

Benchmarks:
1. Measures the effectiveness of documentation tools

2. Trends and quantifies the effectiveness of coding

3. Evaluates the success of concurrent documentation improvement on an ongoing basis

The CDI specialists should have a clinical or health information background with record review experience. They should be effective physician communicators, excellent at reviewing clinical information and data to determine where documentation does not meet the criteria for high quality. Experience with computer programs, data entry, and data analysis is also important. They should be effective trainers. In addition, current or prior experience in the healthcare organization is helpful. Prior experience with clinical documentation training and record review using the criteria for high-quality clinical documentation is ideal. It is likely that many organizations will need to provide initial training to new clinical documentation specialists, so experience and qualifications will be the determining factors in deciding who to hire. The employment interview should be managed as an investigative process. The interviewer(s) should be experienced in CDI management as well as armed with a list of relevant questions (Arvey and Campion 2006). Figure 6.2 is a list of questions that can be used when interviewing candidates for a clinical documentation specialist position.

Health Information and Coding Interface

The goal of every CDI program is to obtain high-quality documentation on a patient's record while the patient is still in house. Some degree of concurrent documentation quality can be obtained through training. The rest of the documentation goal must be achieved by using a record review and query process. An effective program should be able to capture 70 to 75 percent of query responses concurrently. The remainder will need to be obtained

Figure 6.2   Questions for prospective clinical documentation specialists

---

Interview Questions for Prospective Clinical Documentation Improvement Specialists

1. Describe your previous work experience in acute care medicine.

2. Why do you believe you would be a successful documentation improvement specialist? What are your strengths?

3. Describe the various communication skills that you have developed that would make you successful in influencing physicians.

4. How would you handle these scenarios?

    a. The physician rips the query form off the record and throws it into the wastebasket while telling you, "I don't have time for this!"

    b. The physician tells you, "I know this will help the hospital, but what's in it for me?"

    c. A physician tells you, "All this hospital cares about is making more money. That's why they want to make me do this extra work."

    d. After reviewing an elderly woman's record, you see that the patient is diagnosed with pneumonia. The patient is on IV broad spectrum antibiotics and is admitted from the nursing home. The patient is three years status post CVA with mild dysphasia. Based on your expertise as a clinician, you are suspicious that this is a gram negative or aspiration pneumonia. You place a query on the health record asking the physician to be more specific about the type of pneumonia the patient has. The physician states, "The patient is only here for a few days and there is no way I will know what type of pneumonia the patient has. How can you expect me to be more specific?"

---

retrospectively. The most efficient way to capture retrospective queries is through the coding process (Russo 2001). Therefore, it is essential to have the coding staff interfaced with the CDI program staff. The coding staff should understand when there are outstanding concurrent queries upon discharge of the patient. The coding professional should generate a retrospective query to the physician so long as the justification for the query still exists when the patient is discharged. Depending on the program structure, the CDI staff may or may not be directly reporting to the HIM department. Wherever the program reports, the CDI program manager should ensure there is a daily interface between the CDI specialists and the coding staff.

Figure 6.3 illustrates a CDI program structure that shows interface and integration with both the departments of case management and the HIM department. In this example, the CDI function does not report to either function directly, and uses physician liaisons to assist with continuing program interfaces.

Conclusion

Every clinical documentation program must have a structure and support that will ensure its success and sustainability. Program management should include both a physician leader and a CDI manager. Program staffing should be composed, at least initially, of CDI specialists charged with concurrent querying and training, who interface regularly with coding professionals on the retrospective query process. In the ideal structure, the CDI program reports directly to the CMO. In organizations where this direct reporting relationship is not possible, it is still important to ensure that the program reports up through the CMO or that there is a dotted-line reporting relationship between the CDI function and the CMO.

Figure 6.3   Sample clinical documentation improvement organization chart

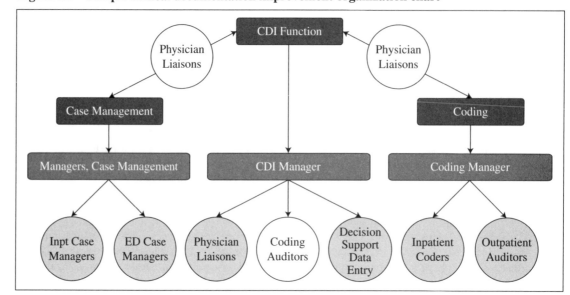

References

Arvey, R. D., and J. E. Campion. 2006. The employment interview: A summary and review of recent research. *Personnel Psychology.* 25(2):281–322.

Grol, R., R. Baker, and F. Moss. 2002. Quality improvement research: Understanding the science of change in health care. *Quality and Safety in Health Care.* 11:110–111.

Keogh, T. and W. Martin. 2004. Managing unmanageable physicians: Leadership, stewardship and disruptive behavior. *Physician Executive.* 30(5):18–22.

Marco, A. P., and D. Buchman. 2003. Influencing physician performance. *Quality Management in Health Care .* 12(1):4–42.

Russo, R. 2001. The application of knowledge management principles to compliant coding activities. *Topics in Health Information Management.* 21(3):18–22.

Russo, R. 2008. *A Compelling Case for Clinical Documentation. Use Clinical Documentation to Achieve Strategic Alignment with Your Medical Staff.* (Volume 1.) Bethlehem, PA: DJ Iber Publishing.

Chapter 7
Physician Training

Introduction

Physician training in high-quality clinical documentation practices is the keystone of every clinical documentation improvement (CDI) program. Clinical documentation training, unfortunately, is not provided to physicians either during medical school or in most residency programs. Therefore, the members of the typical medical staff have had little to no exposure to a formal clinical documentation training program (Cascio et al. 2005). Ideally, every healthcare system or organization involved in training physicians on clinical documentation practices should be using the same program content and methodology for training.

This chapter proposes the use of a scientifically validated method for clinical documentation training known as the CAMP Method. The method draws upon the adult-learning theory of self-efficacy and uses the components of coaching, asking, mastering, and peer learning to teach physicians the principles of high-quality clinical documentation. This method has been statistically proven to produce both higher quality and sustainability of clinical documentation in physician trainees. Moreover, the CAMP Method has been proven to produce significantly more improved documentation results than the traditional type of training provided in most physician CDI training programs. The typical program is defined as one that involves a team consisting of a physician trainer and a clinical documentation expert who lecture physicians for about 45 minutes, using PowerPoint slides and handouts. However, the author has found in her experience with CDI training that many organizations provide even less than the typical 45 minutes of training.

There are three challenges for healthcare organizations in moving forward with a comprehensive physician-training program for clinical documentation. First, the organization must obtain the support of the executive team for such an initiative. The importance of support from the senior management team (and how to obtain it), is addressed in chapter 5 of this book. Second, the organization must identify the appropriate resources for training. Resources include qualified trainers, training materials, and a budget to pay for the training. Third, physicians must attend the training (Parochka and Paprockas 2001). Physician support for the program, including attendance at training sessions, should be the initial responsibility of the executive management team. Ultimately, the physicians must perceive some intrinsic or personal value in the training.

The CAMP Method attempts to demonstrate value for the physicians by using research that is based on the scientific method to support it. Since physicians are trained as scientists and only accept proof of the effectiveness of treatment (or in this case, training) when it has been scientifically proven, they may be more likely to accept training, (such as the CAMP Method) that has been rigorously tested. In addition, the use of the case study method for training and the actual practice of clinical documentation skills during training is an essential part of an effective training program. The CAMP Method uses two 2-hour programs (or four total hours) to train physicians in the core components of high-quality clinical documentation. Each organization will need to assess the value of comprehensive CDI training, like that proposed in the CAMP Method, and determine the best approach for training its medical staff.

Program Instructor

Research has shown that professionals learn best from a peer whom they trust and respect (Bandura 2000). Moreover, if learning from a peer is coupled with coaching, asking, and mastering (described in the methodology section of this chapter), the training will be sustainable. For optimal training outcomes, it is essential for CDI training to be performed by a physician peer. It is also important that the physician trainers be perceived as credible communicators of the training topic. In the case of CDI training, there are few physician experts available to act in that role. Therefore, the best instruction for a physician CDI training program involves a training team. The team should be composed of a physician instructor and a clinical documentation expert. These two individuals, delivering the information together, will likely contribute to an optimal training outcome (Bandura 1986; Lenz and Shortridge-Baggett 2002). The training program for the CAMP Method study was originally conducted with resident physicians at The Hospital of the University of Pennsylvania. The program used a training team with a physician instructor and a clinical documentation expert.

The inclusion of a physician leader for CDI on the team is described in detail in chapter 6, "Staffing the Program". This physician leader can also serve in the training role. If an organization does not have a physician leader on its CDI team initially, it can hire a physician consultant to function in this role in the short term. The key to having an effective training team is including both a clinical documentation expert (to train on content) as well as a physician peer who can share experiences with peers. The physician trainer can also be valuable in managing the physician trainees and assuring them they are capable of practicing high-quality clinical documentation, and it will not involve a significantly greater amount of time than their current practices take.

The nonphysician trainer should be an individual who is well-versed in clinical documentation principles, quality indicators, and coding and reimbursement methodologies. This individual is likely to be an HIM professional or a nurse with the appropriate training in coding and reimbursement. The nonphysician trainer must be comfortable training both small and large groups of physicians and work well with the physician trainer. It is important for the team members to plan their roles in the training process. Table 7.1 contains the ideal and minimum qualifications for a nonphysician trainer. Table 6.2 in chapter 6 shows the ideal and minimum qualifications for the physician leader or trainer.

Table 7.1 Qualifications for nonphysician clinical documentation trainer

Skill	Nonphysician Trainer Ideal	Nonphysician Trainer Minimum
Formal education	Bachelor's degree or above in a clinical area; current licensure or accreditation; academic training in pathophysiology and health information	Bachelor's degree or equivalent with licensure or accreditation in a clinical or healthcare area
Training received in clinical documentation	80 hours or more and certification, if possible	At least 80 hours
Experience in clinical documentation	Experience documenting in patient records; at least five years reviewing documentation in patient records treating patients	At least five years reviewing documentation in patient records
Experience providing classroom instruction	40 hours or more of instruction	At least 40 hours of instruction
Experience providing practical instruction	160 hours of on-unit or in-office observation and feedback	At least 100 hours of on-unit or in-office observation and feedback

Program Attendees

The question of which physicians should attend CDI training must be addressed early in the process. Ideally, all physicians should be responsible for completing basic clinical documentation training. In reality, this may be limited by training capabilities of the organization and the willingness of physicians to participate. The best approach is to prioritize and organize the CDI physician trainees. The exact methodology for prioritizing will vary by organization. Important issues for an organization to consider in identifying the physicians to be trained include the value to the organization and the likelihood of cooperation from the physicians. Using these criteria, the organization should give top priority to the physicians who admit the largest numbers of patients and have historically been cooperative and supportive of organizational initiatives. This may be the organization's hospitalist group or internal medicine physicians. An example of a training plan for a teaching hospital that employs hospitalists is described in the following paragraphs.

Physicians from the hospitalist group are often the top priority for CDI training in many organizations. Hospitalists, who take on the role of the patient's primary care physician when a patient is hospitalized, account for as many as 60 percent of hospital admissions in some hospitals. In other cases, hospitalists account for 100 percent of medical admissions (Wachter and Goldman 2002). Hospitalists should, therefore have a predominant role in CDI training. The training must be carefully balanced with clinical responsibilities because hospitalists carry a very high patient load. Hospitalists, if employed by the organization, can bring value not only in improved inpatient documentation, but also professional-fee documentation (Rifkin 2007).

Residents are often the first-line documenters for inpatient cases. Although they should not be the sole documenters, residents play an important role in any CDI initiative. Programs are most successful if the initial training is provided each year to first-year residents. The organization should clearly define the residents' continuing documentation responsibilities and involve them in years two, three, and four. But, as long as the comprehensive CDI training is provided to each first-year class, by the fourth year of operations, any teaching hospital that adopts this process will have a full complement of residents armed with high-quality clinical documentation skills.

As with hospitalists, residents carry a heavy workload, and current Department of Health and Human Services (HHS) requirements limit the number of hours residents can spend in the hospital in a patient-care role. Training will need to be carefully planned with the director of resident education. An added value of CDI training for the residents is that the training can be used to meet one of the Accreditation Council of Graduate Medical Education (ACGME) competency requirements—the requirement that residents are trained in and familiar with healthcare systems (Barden et al. 2003; Phillbert et al. 2002). Clinical documentation, quality indicators, HIPAA and patient rights, and reimbursement systems, all of which are addressed during the basic CDI program, fulfill this requirement.

Hospital-employed physicians should be a high priority on the CDI training list. If an organization owns any physician practices or employs other physicians within the system, those physicians should be expected to attend CDI training early in the process. Because physician employees of a health system generate documentation related to both hospital care and office-based care, they can begin applying the concepts of high-quality clinical documentation that they learn in the initial training in their office practices. These office practices may also be a good place for eventual expansion of the CDI program beyond the acute care setting (Robinson 1998).

Every hospital has a small group of physicians, usually about 10 to 15 percent of the attending staff, who are responsible for the majority of hospital admissions. These individuals should be identified and targeted for early training. While training can be viewed as a benefit in that it increases a physician's skill set, CDI training should be communicated to the physicians by the hospital's executive team as being a responsibility. This is the message that, in particular, the high-admitting physicians need to hear. Hopefully, because high-admitting physicians have a significant impact on an organization's economic state, the executive team and other managers have positive relationships with them. This makes good business sense and can be used by the CDI program staff in obtaining support from the high-admitting physicians for both attendance at training sessions and overall support for the program.

Members of the medical staff can generally be divided into two groups: those that support new hospital initiatives and those that do not support new hospital initiatives. It is likely that the organization can also identify physicians on either end of this spectrum. There will be about 10 to 15 percent of physicians who are high supporters of any hospital initiative, and who always step up to the plate to help out in any way they can. These physicians should be involved in training as early as possible since they are likely to advocate the value of the training and the program to their peers. This information communication can strengthen program support.

There will also be about 10 to 15 percent of physicians who are strong naysayers of any hospital initiatives. Unfortunately, the negative attitude of these physicians can begin to impact other members of the medical staff. It is important to identify physicians in both of these groups and create a strategy for CDI training. The CDI trainers may need to rely on communications from the CEO and other executive team members to impact the naysayers. The naysayers will be the most difficult group to convert, but the earlier the trainers begin working with them, the greater the positive impact will be for the organization.

Table 7.2 illustrates a sample training schedule for a teaching hospital that employs hospitalists and primary care physicians. Both the physician's time and willingness to participate, as well as training resources, need to be considered when designing the training plan, which should also include a plan for makeup sessions for physicians who cannot attend the initial training.

Table 7.2   Sample 2-year clinical documentation training plan for physicians

Physician

Group	Month																							
	1	2	3	4	5	6	7	8	9	10	11	12	13	14	15	16	17	18	19	20	21	22	23	24
Hospitalists	▓	▓																						
Medicine		▓	▓																					
Medicine specialties			▓	▓																				
General surgeons				▓	▓																			
Surgery specialties					▓	▓																		
OB/GYN Newborn						▓	▓																	
ED Physicians							▓	▓																
Radiologists									▓															
Anesthesiologists				▓	▓																			
Residents	▓			▓	▓																			
Fellows					▓	▓	▓																	
Employed primary care physicians				▓	▓																			
Employed specialists and surgeons			▓	▓	▓																			
Session 1 makeup for medicine specialties										▓	▓													
Session 2 makeup for medicine specialties															▓	▓								
Session 1 makeup for surgical specialties													▓	▓						▓	▓	▓	▓	
Session 2 makeup for surgical specialties																	▓	▓	▓	▓	▓	▓	▓	▓

Methodology

Because the CAMP Method has been proven, through the experimental method, to produce a statistically significant positive difference in clinical documentation quality and sustainability over either traditional training or no training, this is the method that is proposed here (Russo and Fitzgerald 2008). The CAMP acronym stands for the four components used in teaching: coaching, asking, mastering, and peer learning. These components are derived from the theory of self-efficacy, a proven adult-learning model (Bandura 2000; Bandura 1986; Lenz and Shortridge-Baggett 2002) and are briefly described as follows:

- *Coaching* involves reinforcing and encouraging participants about their abilities to perform the function. Here, the physician trainer shares experiences about clinical documentation with the trainees. Coaching should be interactive, and the physician should ask for feedback from the trainees. The physician trainer should be able to manage responses from the trainees so that other physician trainees can benefit from this interactive experience. Essentially, the feedback loop here becomes another form of peer learning.

- *Asking* involves soliciting feedback from the physician participants in a specific manner and at a specific time. At a minimum, the trainers should ask the physicians at the beginning of the program about their concerns regarding the training. This activity can be used to eliminate any misconceptions. It will also reduce or extinguish underlying negativity that may have been harbored by some physicians during the training process. The physician trainer and the nonphysician trainer must be prepared for physician responses and be able to manage these responses to ensure the program proceeds as planned.

- *Mastering* involves practical application of the principles demonstrated and discussed during the training program. Here, physician trainees are given an opportunity to practice high-quality clinical documentation. They are provided with sample health records and case studies, which they are asked individually to review and determine whether the documentation meets the criteria for high-quality clinical documentation. If it does not, then the physician trainees suggest appropriate documentation. The cases are later discussed among the group, which adds to the peer learning component of the training.

- *Peer Learning* involves instruction by a knowledgeable peer. The physician instructor is of prime importance in this component. However, it is also important for the physician trainees to learn from their peers who are also in the program. Soliciting feedback and validating (or correcting) thoughts about the CDI process is an important part of the peer learning process.

The specific use of these components is detailed in table 7.3, which presents the complete agenda used for the CAMP Method study. This can be used as a guide when developing a CDI training program. The agenda refers to questionnaires and tests that the physician trainees were given during the study, but the training can be conducted without these data collection tools. More details about the CAMP Method and survey tools can be found at http://www.acompellingcase.com/.

Table 7.3   Contents of two 2-hour CDI sessions used in the CAMP Method Training First Session

Concept	Activity	Program Design to Incorporate Concept	Time
Peer Learning & Coaching	Introduction	Review session outline and objectives. Physician instructor shares own experience with clinical documentation and assures participants that, with the appropriate training and support, they will master this process.	10 min
Mastering	Self-assessment & test	Participants take the self-assessment and the pre-test; collect the self-assessment and the pre-test from the participants before reviewing the responses.	10 min
Peer Learning	Test review	Review test questions and correct responses with attendees.	10 min
Asking	Physician commitment to good clinical documentation	Discuss the relationship between good documentation practices and improved patient outcomes with the participants. Ask physicians to share their concerns about clinical documentation. Make a list of what the concerns are and share the list (as a way to end this portion of the session). State that we will revisit the list in the second session. Include time management if not addressed by physicians.	10 min
Peer Learning	Documentation rules	Review documentation "rules" PowerPoint with physicians. Ask for and allow questions throughout this portion of the presentation.	15 min
Asking	Break	Serve refreshments and take a 5-minute break.	10 min
Mastering	Case study examples	Review case studies 1–5 that correspond with objectives 2–5.	15 min
Mastering	Tools	Provide each physician with a CDI Handbook and a Pocket Tool for General Medicine. Review the contents of the handbook and the tool. Allow for questions throughout this portion of the presentation.	15 min
Mastering; Coaching	Case study exercises	Give physicians case study exercises 1–5 that contain documentation from actual patient records to review and provide the correct documentation to identify the patient's diagnoses. Review answers with physicians and ask participants for their responses. Provide feedback as participants share their answers.	15 min
Asking	MD Concerns	Revisit list of concerns from beginning of the program.	10 min
Coaching	Conclusion	Conclude the program by assuring the physicians that they can document well. Ask them to apply the concepts they have learned during this session between now and the next session and be prepared to share their experiences during the next session.	5 min
Coaching Peer Learning	Introduction	Review session outline and objectives. Return the pre-test results to each participant. Physician instructor asks participants to share their documentation experiences over the past week. Provide feedback to examples.	15 min
Coaching	Videotape viewing	Have attendees view videotape of physicians. Discuss concerns about documentation. At the completion of the video ask physicians to share their opinions of the documentation concepts shared in the video.	20 min
Mastering; Coaching	Case study examples	Review case studies 6-10 that correspond with objectives 1–6. Ask participants to comment on the examples; Provide feedback on comments.	15 min
Asking	Break	Serve refreshments and take a 5-minute break allowing participants to interact with each other.	10 min

(continued on next page)

Table 7.3   Contents of two 2-hour CDI sessions used in the CAMP Method Training First Session *(continued)*

Concept	Activity	Program Design to Incorporate Concept	Time
Mastering; Coaching	Case study exercises	Give physicians case study exercises 6–10 that contain documentation from actual patient records to review and provide the correct documentation to identify the patients' diagnoses. Review answers with physicians asking participants for their responses. Provide feedback as participants share their answers.	15 min
Mastery; Asking; Coaching	Tools	Ask physicians to refer to their CDI Handbook and Pocket Tool. Ask participants to provide examples of where and when they were able to use the tools over the past week (since the first session). Provide feedback on the use of the tools as shared by the participants. Use any remaining time to review the contents of the book again.	15 min
Asking	Physician commitment	Review listing of concerns generated by residents during previous session. Identify how their dedication and commitment to medicine can be demonstrated through good documentation practices. Ask the residents to sign a "Commitment to Improved Clinical Documentation" form.	10 min
Mastering	Post-test	Have participants take the self-assessment and the post-test. Collect the self-assessments and the post-tests. Review the answers with the participants.	15 min
Coaching	Conclusion	Conclude the program by assuring the physicians that they can document well.	5 min
Coaching; Peer Learning	Evaluation	Ask participants to evaluate the educational program.	2 min

Initial Program Content

Initial program content should focus on the seven criteria for high-quality clinical documentation. These criteria are presented in detail in chapter 1 (can be used in PowerPoint presentations to review with physicians). CDI trainers should use case studies and patient examples from their own organizations to the extent possible. Physician trainees will learn the most from their own documentation experiences. Table 7.4 details the objectives for the keystone training on clinical documentation. Use of these objectives will ensure a thorough and compliant training experience for the organization's medical staff.

Conclusion

Physician training in the principles of high-quality clinical documentation is the most essential component of a CDI program. The main steps in the process are to identify the right team for training, obtain physician support for and attendance at training sessions, design the program content, and teach the program in a manner that will not only increase the quality of clinical documentation, but will also ensure the sustainability of that training.

Table 7.4 Instructional objectives of CDI training program

Overall objective: Following the educational intervention, the physician will demonstrate improved skill in high-quality clinical documentation in patient health records.

Specific objectives: The resident physician will:

1. Demonstrate understanding of the relationship between physician documentation and the translation of that documentation into ICD-9-CM coded data.

2. Demonstrate an understanding that ICD-9-CM coded data is used for planning, reimbursement, quality ratings, Medicare Conditions of Participation, Joint Commission Core Measures, and research.

3. Provide documentation in the inpatient record that is timely, legible, complete, clear, consistent, reliable, and precise.

4. Document detail and precision in the patient's principal diagnosis.

5. Document all chronic coexisting secondary diagnoses.

6. Document all acute coexisting secondary diagnoses.

7. Document the clinical significance of all abnormal diagnostic tests.

8. Document the etiology or suspected etiology of symptoms.

References

Bandura, A. 1986. *Social Foundations of Thought and Action: A Social Cognitive Theory.* Englewood-Cliffs, NY: Prentice-Hall.

Bandura, A. 2000. *Handbook of Principles of Organizational Behavior.* E.A. Locke, ed. Oxford: Blackwell.

Barden, C. B., M. C. Specht, M. D. McCarter, J. M. Daly, and T. J. Fahey. 2003. Effects of limited work hours on surgical training. *Obstetrical and Gynecological Survey.* 58(4):244–245.

Cascio, B. M., J. H. Wilkens, M. C. Ain, C. Toulson, and F. J. Frassica. 2005. Documentation of acute compartment syndrome at an academic healthcare center. *Journal of Bone and Joint Surgery.* 87(2):346.

Lenz, E. R. and L. M. Shortridge-Baggett. 2002. *Self-Efficacy in Nursing: Research and Measurement Perspectives.* New York: Springer Publishing.

Parochka, J. and K. Paprockas, K. 2001. A continuing medical education lecture and workshop, physician behavior, and barriers to change. *Journal of Continuing Education in the Health Professions.* 21(2):10.

Philibert, P., W. T. Friedmann, and N. Williams. 2002. New requirements for resident duty hours. *Journal of the American Medical Association.* 288:1112–1114.

Rifkin, W.D., A. Berger, E.S. Holmboe, and B. Sturdevant. 2007. Comparison of hospitalists and nonhospitalists regarding core measures of pneumonia care. *American Journal of Managed Care.* 13(3):129–132.

Robinson, J.D. 1998. Consolidation of medical groups into physician practice management organizations. *Journal of the American Medical Association.* 279:144–149.

Russo, R. and S. Fitzgerald. 2008. Physician clinical documentation: Implications for healthcare quality and cost. Academy of Management Annual Meeting, Anaheim, CA.

Wachter, R. M., and L. Goldman. 2002. The hospitalist movement 5 years later. *Journal of the American Medical Association.* 287:487–494.

Chapter 8
Training Nonphysician Clinicians and CDI Program Staff

Similar to physician clinical documentation improvement (CDI) training, training for nonphysician clinicians is the keystone of the program. Nonphysician CDI training is divided into training for program staff who may someday teach CDI sessions to clinicians and physicians, and training for nonphysician clinicians who document in patient records. This chapter will begin with the training for CDI program staff, followed by the training for clinicians.

The CAMP Method as described in chapter 7 incorporates the adult-learning theory of self-efficacy, and it uses coaching, asking, mastering, and peer learning to ensure improved quality and sustainability. Although the CAMP Method was tested originally with physicians, it can be used to train anyone (Bandura 2000, 120; Bandura 1986; Lasinger and Tresolini 1999). The primary difference between the format discussed in chapter 7 and the format used for training nonphysician clinicians is in the peer learning component. Peer learning means that trainees are taught by knowledgeable peers who they respect. For instance, if nurses are being trained, then ideally, a nurse would be paired with a clinical documentation expert to deliver the training. Or, if nutritionists are being trained, a nutritionist would be paired with a clinical documentation expert. While it may not always be possible to find a knowledgeable peer, this training team model will produce the optimal outcome for the organization.

Training CDI Program Staff

All CDI program staff should be thoroughly trained in the principles of high-quality clinical documentation as well as the review of patient records to identify possible deficiencies in documentation. Ideally, training will occur as a group. The peer learning component of training is triggered in group settings. This strengthens the sustainability of the training. Group training also ensures consistency of the content being presented.

CDI staff training is a three-part process. The first part involves training the staff in the theory of high-quality clinical documentation. This is similar to the training they will someday provide to physicians and clinicians. This training also involves teaching the basics of coding and the reimbursement process. In the second part, the CDI program staff members are trained in the physician query process. And, finally, they are trained in program data collection and analysis.

Training CDI Staff on the Theory and the Application of CDI

The initial portion of the program on the theory and application of CDI contains the same content as the physician keystone training. Exposure to this training is a good first step for the program staff. It also provides participants with the basis for the physician training program should they ever be on a training team that provides CDI education to physicians.

In addition to the basics, CDI program staff also should be trained on the fundamentals of coding and reimbursement systems. The content in chapter 4 can be referenced to create a more comprehensive training program for the CDI program staff. Finally, because clinical documentation determines both actual and perceived quality of care, it is important for the program staff to be trained on the basics of Medicare quality indicators and to be familiar with public quality report cards like HealthGrades (http://www.healthgrades.com/). Figure 8.1 contains a list of sample training objectives for CDI staff. This sample is specific to the acute care inpatient setting. Training that includes or focuses on outpatient or other inpatient settings would need to be modified to reflect specific objectives.

Figure 8.1   Clinical documentation improvement training program objectives (for the inpatient acute care setting)

1. To adequately prepare the case manager to participate in improving inpatient clinical documentation through record review, application of official guidelines, and interaction with physicians and other clinicians

2. To understand the impact of clinical documentation on severity, mortality, and morbidity "ratings" for inpatient cases

3. To understand the relationship between clinical documentation and case mix index

4. To understand the relationship between clinical documentation and Medicare quality indicators

5. To understand the relationship between clinical documentation and healthcare quality score cards such as HealthGrades (http://www.healthgrades.com) and Joint Commission's Quality Check™ (http://www.jointcommission.org/QualityCheck/06_qc_facts.htm)

6. To identify the correct principal diagnosis statement for inpatient records in every specialty by applying official Uniform Hospital Discharge Data Set (UHDDS) guidelines.

7. To understand the impact that principal diagnosis has on determining the DRG into which the inpatient case is assigned

8. To identify accurate secondary diagnoses for inpatient records in every specialty by applying official UHDDS guidelines

9. To understand the impact that secondary diagnosis documentation has on determining the DRG for the patient's acute inpatient stay

10. To identify opportunities in the health record where clinical documentation could be further clarified to result in capturing more specific principal diagnoses

11. To identify opportunities in the health record where clinical documentation could be further clarified to result in capturing more specific or additional secondary diagnoses

12. To identify opportunities in the health record where clinical documentation could be further clarified to result in capturing more specific procedures

13. To formulate a valid concurrent physician query

Training CDI Staff on the Record Review and Query Process

The primary operational components of the CDI program are the record review and the query process. It is the review process and the physician query process that allow for the highest level of quality in clinical documentation. Therefore, training on both the record review and query process should be part of the CDI program staff training. Classroom training should consist of the theoretical basis for the program, the appropriate way to review a record to identify documentation deficiencies, and the parameters for querying a physician. When the classroom training is about 50 percent complete, the CDI program staff members can begin to visit the nursing units, and begin to review health records and apply the initial information they have learned. During this initial review of records on the units, the CDI program participants should be paired with an experienced CDI specialist. Ideally, a CDI staff trainee receives feedback about the review process and learns to identify query opportunities. This on-unit review progresses until the CDI staff trainee begins to query physicians. The CDI staff trainee should be observed and given feedback until the trainer witnesses accurate record review and appropriate, consistent querying. CDI staff trainees generally need about 40 to 50 hours of observation before they can function independently.

The record review process should include addressing all components of the patient record as possible sources for query opportunities. The clinical indicators and clinical evidence in sample records should be reviewed with the trainees, preferably by the physician leader for CDI. It is important to have the physician leader involved in this process, as opposed to a CDI peer because of the perspective the physician brings. CDI staff benefit from continuous exposure to the physician's perspective throughout their training. This interaction better prepares the CDI staff member for the one-on-one physician query process that is the keystone of the program. It is important that the CDI staff trainee can identify any documentation in a patient record that does not meet the criteria for high-quality clinical documentation. Every documentation deficiency presents a possible opportunity for a physician query.

The physician query process should be explained initially in the classroom setting. Role playing between the CDI trainees and the physician leader for CDI is helpful before attempting a live query on the nursing unit. The query process can be a live verbal query or a written query. Regardless of how a query is generated, it should be clearly captured in the program documentation. More detail about the query process is addressed in chapter 9.

Training CDI Staff on the Data Collection Process

It has been said that if you cannot measure a process, you cannot manage it. This is true for all activities, including clinical documentation. Therefore, CDI program staff should be trained on the collection of program data, entering data elements into the program database, following up on unanswered queries, and identifying trends using program data. The following sections will review each of these activities separately.

The collection of program data includes the identification of:

1. All cases that were reviewed

2. The number of cases with queries

3. The nature of the query

4. The physician's response to the query

These primary data elements are the basis for reporting the key metrics of the program. The key metrics of the program, which are determined by the senior management of the organization (and discussed in chapter 10), determine program success and the likelihood that the organization will continue to support a clinical documentation program.

The program staff members are responsible for entering the data elements into the program database. Several viable options are available for collecting CDI program data. Some organizations use case management software that has been modified for CDI purposes. Most programs use software that can be licensed from one of the consulting firms that offers clinical documentation services, like Navigant Consulting. The Navigant software, known as the CDI Monitor, allows the input of a significant amount of program data and then generates reports using these data elements. The CDI staff must be thoroughly trained on the appropriate use of the software to ensure accurate program reporting. Once trained, data input should be reviewed during the course of the first month to ensure acceptable quality. Figure 8.2 shows a CDI Monitor data entry form for a record that has been reviewed or queried. Ideally, the CDI specialist enters this information directly into the computer. However, for organizations that do not have wireless laptops available to the CDI specialists, the CDI form can be used.

Post-training Evaluation

The entire training program for CDI staff will likely be a 60- to 80-hour process. After training has been completed, all CDI specialists should be tested on their knowledge and skill level. The testing instrument serves as evidence of what the CDI specialist has learned. It also serves as evidence of areas where there are gaps in knowledge. So, an organization must follow up on any knowledge or skill gaps as soon as they are identified. In addition to testing, it is helpful to have the CDI specialists perform a self-evaluation. Research has shown that self-evaluations such as the one in figure 8.3 are often as good an indicator of knowledge and skill gaps as testing instruments. This type of evaluation takes only a few minutes for the program staff to complete and can provide information that can help improve both the program and the training process.

Figure 8.3 shows a CDI specialist self-evaluation that can be used to measure the improvements provided by training as well as the existing gaps in knowledge.

Training Nonphysician Clinicians

Every clinician who documents in a patient record should receive at least initial training in CDI. Furthermore, clinicians who are well trained on the clinical documentation process may have a positive influence on physicians' documentation practices. At a minimum, trained clinicians' documentation can be used to generate clinically-validated queries. While this seems like a simple statement, implementation of the task can be difficult. The best way to accomplish this training is to communicate the basics of the CDI program to all clinical managers and with their input create a thorough schedule for training.

Figure 8.2.   CDI Monitor data entry form

CDI Monitor Data Record
Prepared by Navigant Consulting, Inc. for

Medical Record

Encounter #:		Physician:	
Medical Record #:		Facility:	
Patient Name:		Insurance:	

DRG Assignment

CDS Name	Admit Date	CDS Review Date	Working DRG	CDS DRG

Coder Name	Discharge Date	Coder DRG	Final DRG

Queries

CDS or Coder	Date	Physician	Response*	Response Date	Query**

Notes

Query Listing:

Abnormal Labs	Abnormal Tests	AMI Secondary Diagnosis	Anemia - Medical
Anemia - Surgical	Cardiac Cath. secondary Conditions	Carotid Stenosis	Cerebral Infarction
Chest Pain	Consultation Agreement	CVA - Infarction	Diabetic Manifestations
Documentation Clarification	Malnutrition	More Acute Conditions	Pneumonia
Renal Failure	Respiratory Failure	Secondary Conditions	Sepsis
Severity of Illness	Surgical Conditions	Surgical Debridement	Symptoms

Documentation Specialist Information on this form is to be used for documentation improvement purposes only. Any coding or DRG assignment is for draft or working purposes only and is not to be used for final coding or billing purposes. The coder assigns the final DRG.
* Possible responses: Awaiting/Yes/No/No Response.

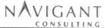

Page 1 of 1

Figure 8. 3   CDI specialist self-evaluation

DOCUMENTATION IMPROVEMENT PROGRAM										

CDI Specialist Self-Evaluation

Directions: Please complete the following statements by indicating your level of knowledge and familiarity with the concepts addressed BEFORE the start of the documentation improvement program as well as your knowledge CURRENTLY of the same concepts. Circle the number which best represents your level of knowledge and familiarity both before and currently. "1" signifies no knowledge and "5" represents a strong knowledge of the concept.

My knowledge of:	Before Training					After Training				
	Weak				Strong	Weak				Strong
1. The relationship between documentation & coding	1	2	3	4	5	1	2	3	4	5
2. The relationship between coding & reimbursement	1	2	3	4	5	1	2	3	4	5
3. General logic of the DRG Systems	1	2	3	4	5	1	2	3	4	5
4. A patient's principal diagnosis	1	2	3	4	5	1	2	3	4	5
5. The role of secondary diagnoses	1	2	3	4	5	1	2	3	4	5
6. Case mix index (CMI)	1	2	3	4	5	1	2	3	4	5
7. The importance of the *physician* documenting a patient's condition	1	2	3	4	5	1	2	3	4	5
8. The need for physicians to document the significance of lab/other test results	1	2	3	4	5	1	2	3	4	5
9. How pneumonia is categorized in the DRG system	1	2	3	4	5	1	2	3	4	5
10. The difference between reimbursement for COPD vs. respiratory failure	1	2	3	4	5	1	2	3	4	5
11. The impact that secondary diagnoses can make on the reimbursement for acute MI patients	1	2	3	4	5	1	2	3	4	5
12. The importance of identifying the etiology for symptoms, if known	1	2	3	4	5	1	2	3	4	5
13. The importance of documenting differential diagnoses for symptoms with uncertain etiology	1	2	3	4	5	1	2	3	4	5
14. The reimbursement principle that requires the coding of any condition that a physician documents as "possible," "probable," or "questionable" as though the condition exists	1	2	3	4	5	1	2	3	4	5
15. The relationship between physician documentation and healthcare report cards (HealthGrades)	1	2	3	4	5	1	2	3	4	5
16. The relationship between physician documentation and Medicare quality indicators	1	2	3	4	5	1	2	3	4	5
17. The physician query process	1	2	3	4	5	1	2	3	4	5
I would like to know more about:										
Other comments:										

Who Needs to be Trained?

Every clinician who documents in the patient's record should receive CDI training. One way to determine all of these positions in an organization is to review 10 to 20 health records and identify every clinician (by title, not by name) who has documented in the record. Chances are great that a review of a sample of records will identify an exhaustive listing of clinicians for training purposes.

Once the clinicians have been identified, the training should be scheduled. As with physician training, the best way to begin is by obtaining support from the clinicians' leader. The department manager or director should be informed about the CDI education well in advance of any scheduling occurring. Because, it is important to include a peer learning component in the training, the manager is often the best person to help identify who that peer instructor might be.

Because all staff cannot be trained concurrently due to clinicians' schedules and the organization's training capacity, it is important to create a training schedule. Priorities can be set based on criteria such as training clinicians whose documentation is most likely to be relied upon for querying and training clinicians who document the most in patient records.

The first criteria, clinicians whose documentation is likely to be relied upon for querying, may focus on midlevel practitioners. In fact, physician assistants and nurse practitioners should be given high priority for training because of their partnership with physicians. Following is a list of clinicians who should be trained in the basics of high-quality clinical documentation.

- Physician assistants

- Nurse practitioners

- Nurses

- Nutritionists

- Respiratory therapists

- Physical therapists

- Occupational therapists

- Case managers

- Social workers and discharge planners

Who Should Do the Training?

Training should be provided by a team. The best results will come from a program taught by a clinical documentation expert paired with a peer of the group that is being trained. This may not always be feasible, but when possible, peer learning should be used. Preparation for the peer learning process can be done by identifying one key member from each clinical group that will be trained. These individuals may receive some training with the CDI specialists or one-on-one training and feedback on the nursing units. They will not become documentation experts immediately but they should know enough to explain the basic concepts to their peers. The use of a peer trainer increases the sustainability of the training and is a good investment for the organization (Ford-Gilboe et al. 1997; Goldenberg et al. 2005; Opacic 2003).

What Should Be Trained?

The best approach is to train the clinicians using the same content as for the physician training. This is helpful because it exposes the clinicians to all of the fundamental concepts. In addition, it gives the clinicians the opportunity to become familiar with the same training process that the physicians underwent (Bandura 2000, 120). If clinicians should have the opportunity to discuss a clinical documentation practice with a physician, they can refer back to the training as a common point of reference.

Conclusion

In addition to training physicians and CDI program staff, it is essential to train all clinicians who document in patient records. The clinicians and CDI program staff should be trained using the same CAMP Method concepts that were used to train physicians, and they should also be trained on the same basic content. The CDI program staff should participate in a three-part training process to achieve maximum results. When training nonphysician clinicians, to the extent possible, peer learning should be used. When peer clinicians are trained initially and intensively in CDI, their assistance during the training session should result in increased sustainability of the program.

References

Bandura, A. 1986. *Social Foundations of Thought and Action: A Social Cognitive Theory*. Englewood-Cliffs, NY: Prentice-Hall.

Bandura, A. 2000. E.A. Locke, ed. *Handbook of Principles of Organizational Behavior*. Oxford: Blackwell.

Ford-Gilboe, M., H. S. Laschinger, Y. Laforet-Fliesser, C. Ward-Griffin, and S. Foran. 1997. The effect of a clinical practicum on undergraduate nursing students' self-efficacy for community-based family nursing practice. *Journal of Nursing Education*. 36(5):212–220.

Goldenberg, D., M. Andrusyszn, D. Iwasiw. 2005. The effect of classroom simulation on nursing students' self-efficacy related to health teaching. *Journal of Nursing Education*. 44(7):310.

Laschinger, H. K., and C. Tresolini. 1999. An exploratory study of nursing and medical students health promotion counseling self-efficacy. *Nurse Education Today*. 19(5):408–418.

Opacic, D.A. 2003. The relationship between self-efficacy and student physician assistant clinical performance. *Journal of Allied Health*. 32(3):158.

Chapter 9
Documentation Review and Physician Queries

The core operational components of a clinical documentation program are concurrent documentation review and physician queries. The documentation review occurs concurrently with the patient's stay, or as close in time to the patient's treatment and care as possible. The purpose of documentation review is to identify any documentation that does not meet the criteria for high-quality clinical documentation and to ask the physician who authored the documentation to clarify the entry. Ideally, all physicians in an organization should be trained on the principles of clinical documentation.

The activity of querying physicians has been a common practice for the past two decades. Initially, physician querying was performed only by coding professionals in the health information management department. Based on the need to obtain accurate documentation for coding purposes, coding professionals would complete a written query form and ask the physician to clarify certain documentation in the record. Coding is a primary reason for high-quality clinical documentation in the patient health record. However, as discussed throughout the book, healthcare quality report cards, quality of care, and patient satisfaction are three additional, equally important reasons. This chapter will address the concurrent documentation review and establishing metrics for this process, specific problematic documentation, and the physician query process. A key resource for the physician query process that should be used by every CDI program is the AHIMA practice brief entitled, "Managing an Effective Query Process" (AHIMA 2008).

Setting Program Targets and Goals

In order to be both effective and efficient, every CDI operation must be guided by policies, procedures, and key metrics, which are expectations regarding productivity (Curtright et al. 2000). In a CDI program, the activities that should be guided and measured are record review and the query process. As with any decision-making process, clinical documentation policies and measures should be developed specifically by and for each organization. Generic policies and measures can be used as a guide. However, to ensure alignment between the policy, procedure, measures, and the probability that staff in the organization will use them effectively, every document and decision should be customized for the organization.

Establishing and Tracking the Concurrent Record Review Rate

While a 100 percent concurrent documentation review rate is desirable, for most organizations is it unrealistic. The reasons for this are two-fold. First, today about 10 percent of inpatient cases are one-day stays, which makes it difficult to perform any meaningful review. Second, most organizations do not have staffing to cover a 100 percent review of all cases, even if one-day stays are excluded from the inpatient population. It is important to determine an achievable review rate for the organization—one that the staff can work to meet.

A valid, target review rate is determined through the assessment process and some trial and error. The concurrent review portion of the assessment process, addressed in chapter 4, should have established an initial concurrent review rate. However, this rate is just a snapshot in time and the rate will need to be validated. Many organizations take one to three months during or after program implementation to determine a valid review rate. This requires data to be collected carefully on a daily basis. The number of records reviewed by each CDI specialist should be collected and compared over time to determine an average valid rate. Because the program is just in its beginning stages, productivity will be lower than after the staff members have been able to refine their skills over time. Therefore, during the first year, it is a good idea to continue to validate the review rates and to periodically "raise the bar" to ensure expectations are high enough to keep staff members motivated—but so high as to discourage them.

Establishing and Tracking the Query Rate

The same process for determining an organization-specific, record-concurrent review rate should be used to determine the query rate. Initial data from the assessment will provide a good basis. Over time program staff members continue to validate the target rates. Tracking the query rate is important because it can help determine whether the program is achieving its goals. For example, if the initial query rate is set at a 35 percent target, but by the end of the second year of the program, the query rate is 40 percent, this may be evidence that the program is not working effectively. Unless there is a specific reason for an increase, such as a new group of physicians that has not yet been trained in documentation principles, there is reason for concern, and the organization should consider a program re-assessment by an external organization. With continued querying and follow-up training, query rates should decrease over time.

With the expected decrease in query rate, should an organization expect to decrease program staff? No, the staff should not be decreased. Rather, the focus should be shifted to more intensive follow-up training to lower the query rate even further. The focus can also move to other areas of the organization where the CDI program has not yet penetrated. Once an organization has a trained team of CDI specialists, the value of these individuals to the organization is high as long as the organization uses their skills strategically.

Both overall and individual query rates can also be used to identify potential issues with training. For example, if the overall query rate is meeting the target of a 30 percent query rate, but five staff members are querying at a 35 percent query rate and one staff member is querying at a 24 percent query rate, these numbers may show the need for additional training for one or all of the staff members. In addition, if the query rate is significantly lower than the target, and the target rate has been validated, staff members may need additional one-on-one query training on the nursing units. The process of observing staff members and providing feedback about the query process can be an effective training tool.

The query rate is calculated by dividing the number of records that were queried by the total number of records reviewed. So, if 100 records are reviewed, and of that group, 30 records contain queries, the query rate is 30 percent. Data collection can be manual or electronic, although electronic collection is preferred for reliability and preservation of CDI data over time. The process for collecting information should be well organized prior to the actual implementation of the program.

Establishing and Tracking the Query Response Rate

Establishing and tracking the query response rate is different from establishing the review and query rates because there is an additional component. The response rate here depends on the physician who is being queried. If the physician responds, the query response rate goes up, if the physician does not respond, the response rate goes down. In the chapter on program vision, we discussed the importance of an organization's executive team obtaining the initial support from physicians. Other factors that may play a role in physician cooperation include whether the physicians attended training and how they scored on post-testing (if they were tested).

The mechanics of the CDI program and the timing of the patient's discharge can also impact the query response rate. The mechanics of the program determine how a rate is calculated. The query response rate is calculated by dividing the number of responses by the number of queries. So, if 50 queries are issued and 25 physicians respond to them, the response rate is 50 percent. However, this number can vary based upon the program's definition of "response to a query." For example, if the CDI program requires the query be responded to within 24 hours of the query being asked, it will have a different result than if it requires the query to be responded to within 48 hours of the query being asked. In addition, it is important to determine how the calculation will address short-stay patients or queries that are asked the day prior to discharge. If the program allows physicians 36 hours versus 24 hours after discharge to respond to a query, the response rate will vary.

Every organization must determine the definition of a physician response and exactly how the response rate will be calculated. While there is no industry benchmark for this calculation yet, the documentation is essential to accurate coding and organizations may want to consider using the same timeframe for query responses as they use for final coding. For example, if a hospital's policy is to drop bills within 72 hours of final discharge, then the physician query response should be consistent with this policy. Without a standard, well-documented approach, it is not possible to compare rates over time. Physicians should be informed about the timeframe in which they have to respond. It is the CDI program's responsibility to ensure that if a physician is queried on a patient record just prior to the patient's discharge, the physician is adequately informed of that query, for instance via e-mail or a messaging system embedded in the EHR (AHIMA 2008). Whatever the communication mechanism that is used to inform physicians about outstanding queries, it must be reliable and consistent. The physicians must be aware of how they will be informed of outstanding queries and what their responsibility is to respond.

Establishing and Tracking a Query Validation or Agreement Rate

This last key operations metric is important to establish because it measures the degree to which the physicians and the CDI program staff are synchronized in their understanding of the query and CDI process. In addition, this metric can be used to show that the organization does not have an expectation that physicians will respond to every query by documenting an additional diagnosis or additional information about a patient's diagnosis in the record. Sometimes, the documentation is valid as originally entered, but the physician just needs to confirm the documentation. For example, the physician documents the patient's diagnosis as chest pain. The CDI specialist queries the physician for a diagnosis or etiology of the chest pain. The physician may respond with documentation in the progress note, "chest pain, etiology undetermined." In this case, there would be a lack of agreement by the physician that the symptom had an etiology (as asked by the CDI specialist). Another example would be for a patient with several laboratory tests with low potassium levels. The query asks the physician to document the diagnosis represented by the abnormal laboratory tests. The physician documents, "K levels within normal limits for this patient with CHF." This is another example of the physician not agreeing with the question that asks for a diagnosis to represent the abnormal laboratory values (IPRO 2005a).

It is important to collect the agreement rate because if it is too high or too low, it may represent a more systemic problem with the documentation process. For example, if the agreement rate is 100 percent, the physician is agreeing with the CDI specialist on all queries. This may be evidence of either leading queries or physicians who were not properly trained in clinical documentation practices. If the query agreement rate is too low, it may indicate that unnecessary queries are being asked. Or, it may represent problems with physician documentation that can be easily corrected with additional training. The chest pain and low potassium level documentation examples could be corrected through focused physician follow-up education.

Table 9.1 shows an organization's key metrics. In each case, the organization set a target. The table indicates the actual rates for the quarter as well as the percentage of achievement for that metric. Physician response rates appear to be the biggest concerns for this organization.

The Importance of Concurrent Record Reviews

Obtaining clinical documentation in a patient's record while the patient is being tracked (or concurrent with treatment and care) has been shown to produce higher quality of care (Cascio et al. 2005). In addition, the physician's memory of the patient and the actual treatment interaction is clearer during the treatment as opposed to days or weeks after the patient has been discharged. While there is no specific regulatory guideline that limits when a physician can be queried to provide documentation clarification in a patient's record, every organization should develop a policy to address this issue. The primary goal for all CDI programs should be to obtain complete documentation in the patient's record prior to discharge.

The CDI staff's concurrent record review should occur on the second day of admission. All clinical documentation present in the patient's record should be assessed to determine if there are any occurrences where the criteria for high-quality clinical documentation has not been met. If a documentation deficiency exists, the CDI specialist should generate a query, notify the physician, and record the query in the program data base. If the record does not contain any deficiencies, the CDI specialist should record the review in the program data base. For every record reviewed, whether a query was generated or not, the CDI specialist should record the date for follow-up review in the program database (or manual tickler file if the program does not use an electronic data collection tool). The follow-up review should be one to two days from the initial review.

Table 9.1   Sample clinical documentation key measures

Key Metric	Quarter 1	Target*	% Achievement
Concurrent: Record review rate	75%	90%	83%
Concurrent: Physician **query** rate	40%	40%	100%
Physician **response** rate	50%	75%	67%
Physician **validation** rate	70%	80%	88%
Retrospective: Physician **query** rate	5%	15%	33%
Physician **response** rate	100%	60%	60%
Physician **validation** rate	65%	85%	76%

*Note: Targets are not suggested. The targets noted were created specifically by the healthcare organization using its own assessment data. All targets should be organization-specific and be validated on at least an annual basis.

Physician Queries

A physician query can be defined as a question that is directed to a physician and is asked to obtain clarification of documentation in a patient's record when the current documentation does not meet one or more of the criteria for high-quality clinical documentation. Therefore, the patient's record must contain clinical evidence to support any questions (or queries) that are being asked to the physician regarding documentation in that record. The physician query process should be well documented with a written policy and procedure for each organization. The query should clearly identify for the physician the clinical evidence in the record that is prompting the query. All staff members who are involved in querying physicians, as well as the physicians, should be trained on the query process. Some important elements that are found in the AHIMA practice briefs, quality improvement organization (QIO) statements regarding clinical documentation, and in the CMS guidelines include the following (AHIMA 2008; IPRO 2005a; IPRO 2005b; CMS 2006):
Queries should only be asked:

1. If there is valid clinical evidence that the documentation is incomplete or does not meet one of the seven criteria for high-quality clinical documentation

2. By an individual with solid clinical knowledge

3. In an open-ended manner (physicians must document a response and cannot just respond yes or no)

4. In a nonleading manner (without pointing physicians to a specific response)

5. To the individual whose documentation is in question or who is responsible for interpreting test results and other data in the patient's record

Every organization should develop a query policy and procedure that is specific to its organization and that addresses:

1. When queries will be asked

2. Who will ask queries and to whom queries will be asked

3. The hospital's responsibility in supporting the query process

4. The physician's responsibility in responding to queries

5. Acceptable ways to respond to queries

The organization will also want to ensure the physicians have access to the record. In addition, a standard format for the query form should be delineated. Finally, the organization should establish whether the form will be an approved, permanent document in the health record or whether an addendum is required. In every case, a physician's response should be incorporated into the health record. If the form is to become a part of the health record, hospital policies and medical staff bylaws must support this practice.

While the seven criteria for high-quality clinical documentation provide an objective basis for generating a query, it is helpful for an organization to provide examples of when a physician query is required. Conversely, examples of when a physician query is not required should also be addressed. Often, cases where a query should not be generated involve physician documentation of a clinical condition that is not supported by the evidence in the record. This scenario is one that requires a peer review, not a query from the CDI specialist or a coding professional. Examples of when a query is required may include the following:

1. Documentation of reportable conditions or procedures is conflicting, ambiguous, or is otherwise incomplete.

2. Abnormal diagnostic test results indicate the possible addition of a secondary diagnosis or higher specificity of an already documented condition.

3. The patient is receiving treatment for a condition that has not been documented.

4. Abnormal operative or procedural findings are not documented.

5. It is unclear as to whether a condition was ruled out.

6. The principal diagnosis (the reason, after study, for admission) is not clearly identified (AHIMA 2008; IPRO 2005a; IPRO 2005b).

Figure 9.1 is an example of a query policy and procedure developed for an academic medical center. The policy is specific to the needs and processes of the organization. It can be used as an example, but in order for a policy and procedure to be effective for an organization, it must be one that is organization specific.

Specific Problematic Documentation

Due to the compliance concerns surrounding the possible leading queries, CMS has engaged the QIOs to assist in record review for certain targeted DRG and documentation concerns. The reviews are performed as part of the Hospital Payment Monitoring Program (HPMP). They are selected and updated by CMS on an annual basis using historical knowledge and experience related to medically unnecessary admissions, inappropriate readmissions, and diagnosis-related group (DRG) incorrect coding. Some of the specific problematic documentation includes documentation for sepsis and related conditions, pneumonia, congestive heart failure, and blood loss anemia. The documentation for sepsis and related conditions is addressed in detail below and provides an example of the level of detail that HPMP information should be made available to the CDI staff. Often QIO training and communications are directed to the HIM or finance departments in the hospital. It is essential that the CDI function be included in all communications from the QIO.

Figure 9.1   Sample query policy and procedure

Retrospective queries—HIM coders will query the patient's MD if opportunities to improve documentation are noted during retrospective review of the patient's record. Queries of the attending physician after discharge should be made only when there is sufficient supporting documentation within the body of the health record to warrant a query. Questions about documentation in the record may arise during the coding process or as a result of a special audit.

The physician will be queried in the following situations:

1. Documentation is inconsistent and or ambiguous, unclear, incomplete, unspecified. or general in nature (AHIMA Standards of Ethical Coding and Compliance Guidance for Third Party Billing Companies 1999)
2. Principal diagnosis (reason for admission, after study) is not clearly identified
3. Significant CID Specialist queries not answered prior to discharge (those which would impact severity level)
4. Abnormal diagnostic test results indicate the possible addition of a secondary diagnosis or increased specificity of an already documented condition
5. Lack of clarity as to whether a condition has been ruled out
6. Patient is receiving treatment for a condition that has not been documented
7. Significance of abnormal operative, procedural, or pathologic findings is not documented
8. Predetermined and agreed upon (with medical staff) clinical criteria are not met
9. Agreement and documentation of diagnoses documented by other members of the health care team (nutrition, substance abuse team [if not completed by MD member of team], wound care team) needs need physician verification

Query format

The physician query form will be used for all queries, including patient identification, reason for query, directions as to how to provide the requested documentation clarification, and contact information of the person executing the query. When there are multiple questions for one case, the physician is to be alerted that there is more than one query requiring a response.

1. In completing the reason for query on the physician query form, the coder will use open-ended questions and allow the physician to render and document the clinical interpretation of the diagnosis, condition, or procedure, based on the facts of the case. Closed-ended or leading questions will be avoided.
2. Exceptions to the open-ended query, when it is appropriate to query for a specific diagnosis, include the following:
   a. Positive lab or radiology findings clinically supporting the diagnosis (*Coding Clinic*, 2nd quarter. 1998)
   b. Medication is prescribed that supports the specific diagnosis (*Coding Clinic*, 1st quarter, 1993, 2nd quarter, 1998)
3. Physicians (attending or resident) are to respond to retrospective queries within five business days and for special audits, on the same day.
4. If physicians agree with the query, they are to document on a form. (All entries must be signed and dated for the date the current entry is made.)
5. If physicians disagree with the query, they are to indicate the reasons on the physician query form and return the form to the HIM department.

The form shall be documented by the physician and scanned into the hospital's imaging system, if the physician documents additional information.

Sepsis or Urosepsis?

The terms sepsis or urosepsis may be documented by a physician when a more detailed condition is actually present and clinically supported. In most cases, had the physician been trained in the nuances of some of the diagnostic details, the entry would have been documented differently. The QIOs (quality improvement organizations) have created excellent tools to assist hospitals in training physicians, coding professionals, and clinical documentation staff. The definitions below for sepsis, septicemia, and related conditions are from IPRO, the New York State QIO, and the Texas QIO (TMF). Each definition provides clinical information that CDI specialists can use to help determine whether to query physicians. Each condition will result in different ICD-9-CM coding and may result in a different DRG assignment as well.

Septicemia

- A systemic disease with the presence and persistence of pathogenic microorganisms or toxins in the blood (such as viruses, bacteria, fungus, or other organisms)

- Septicemia and sepsis are no longer considered synonymous

Sepsis

- Sepsis = systemic inflammatory response syndrome (SIRS)

- Sepsis is SIRS due to infection. Infection can originate anywhere in the body and be triggered by a bacterial, viral, parasitic, or fungal infection

Severe Sepsis

- SIRS due to infection with organ dysfunction

- Sepsis associated with acute dysfunction in one or more organs

- Organ dysfunction may be cardiovascular, renal, respiratory, hepatic, hematological, central nervous system, or metabolic acidosis

SIRS

- SIRS is the systemic response to infection or trauma

- The systemic response is manifested by a variety of clinical signs and symptoms such as:

    —Fever (temperature) >38 degrees C (100.4 degrees F)

    —Hypothermia <36 degrees C (96.8 degrees F)

    —WBC > or equal to 12000 cells/mm3 (leukocytosis)

    —WBC < or equal to 4000 cells/mm3 (leukopenia) or 10 percent immature cells (bands)

    —Heart rate >90 beats per minute (tachycardia)

    —Respirations >20 breaths per minute or a PcCO2 <32 milligrams of mercury

—Hypotension

—Altered mental status (comatose, confused, lethargy, obtunded)

Septic Shock

- Sepsis with hypotension or a failure of the cardiovascular system

- Endotoxic shock and gram negative shock are synonymous with septic shock

- Septic shock = severe sepsis

Bacteremia

- Bacteria in the blood without an associated inflammatory response

- Denotes laboratory findings of viable bacteria in the blood with no systemic manifestations

- Progresses to septicemia only when there is a more severe infectious process or an impaired immune system

Urosepsis

- Infection confined to the urinary system

- Refers to pyuria or bacteria in the urine (not in the blood)

- Query the physician to determine if the bacteria in the urine has progressed to septicemia or sepsis (IPRO 2005b).

Other Problematic Documentation

Other diagnoses that have been identified by CMS as problematic for complete and accurate documentation include blood loss anemia, congestive heart failure, and pneumonia. The concern by CMS in some cases may also be that the physician has documented a condition, such as blood loss anemia, without the accompanying clinical criteria for blood loss anemia being met. In these cases, the QIO's will determine that the diagnosis was not a valid one and deny payment to the hospital. Every hospital can prevent this type of occurrence through proper physician training, referral of such documentation problems to peer review (or the physician CDI leader), and with close review and incorporation of all HPMP communications into the physician training and query processes.

Retrospective Review

Retrospective review in most organizations will be performed by the coding staff during the coding process. At this time, the coding professionals can determine whether there is an opportunity for a valid physician query based on the clinical evidence in the patient's record. In addition, when there are outstanding physician queries from the concurrent review, the coding professionals can and should follow up on those queries. Retrospective review and querying serves as a safety net to the CDI program and is a process that enables a coding professional to translate physician documentation into coded data with the highest possible accuracy. As noted in the key metric examples at the beginning of the chapter, the retrospective query rate should be much lower than the concurrent query rate; no more than 10 percent. If the retrospective query rate is higher than 10 to 15 percent, it may be evidence of the need for additional physician training and increased productivity or training for the CDI program staff. In addition, the physician response rate for retrospective queries should be 100 percent (UVA 2008). If possible, hospitals should work with the medical staff to include outstanding queries as an incomplete health record deficiency for which a physician's admission privileges can be suspended. Given the importance of the most accurate documentation, both administration and medical staff members should support such a policy.

Teaming Clinical Documentation and Coding Professionals

CDI staff and coding professionals can be teamed to achieve organizational CDI goals. Some of the ways that organizations can team CDI staff and coding professionals include:

1. Involve the coding staff in the initial CDI specialist training

2. Have coding managers and staff train CDI specialists on the coding and reimbursement systems

3. Train coding and CDI staff together on the use of the CDI program database. In most cases, both groups will be entering data into the database for queries. CDI specialists will use the database to enter concurrent reviews and queries, and coding professionals will use it to enter retrospective queries.

4. Have monthly meetings to discuss current QIO initiatives and communications and to analyze program data that may help both CDI and coding staff understand where continued documentation problems are and which physicians appear to have the most significant problems

5. Invite coding professionals to attend physician follow-up training sessions

6. Pair each CDI specialist with a coding professional to track the final resolution of outstanding concurrent queries at the time the patient is discharged

7. Charge the coding staff with specific focus on one or two-day-stay cases where CDI program staff are unable to generate a concurrent query. These cases can also be shared between CDI and coding partners to review for query opportunities as soon as the patient is discharged.

Conclusion

The physician concurrent query process is the core operational component of every CDI program. The process should be clearly explained in organization-specific policies and procedures. These policies and procedures should be documented, updated on at least an annual basis and made available for any physician, manager, or relevant staff member to review. Both physicians and program staff should be thoroughly trained on the query process. The organization should develop key metrics with organization-specific target rates. These rates should be developed using initial assessment and actual day-to-day operations data. In addition, the targets should be reviewed and validated on at least an annual basis.

References

AHIMA. 2008. Managing an effective query process. *Journal of AHIMA*. 79(10): 83–88.

Cascio, B. M., J. H. Wilkens, M. C. Ain, C. Toulson, and F. J. Frassica. 2005. Documentation of acute compartment syndrome at an academic healthcare center. *Journal of Bone and Joint Surgery*. 87 (2):346.

Centers for Medicare and Medicaid Services (CMS) and the National Center for Health Statistics (NCHS). 2006. ICD-9-CM Official Guidelines for Coding and Reporting. www.cdc.gov/nchs/datawh/ftpserv/ftpicd9/ftpicd9.htm.

Curtright, J.W., S.C. Stolp-Smith, E.S. Edell. (2000). Strategic performance management: Development of a performance measurement system at the Mayo Clinic. *Journal of Healthcare Management*. 45 (1):58-68.

IPRO. 2005a. Coding for Quality: Documentation Tips for the Top Seven DRGs. Revised 2005, Hospital Payment Monitoring Program. http://providers.ipro.org/index/hpmp.

IPRO. 2005b. Coding for Quality: Documentation Tips for the Top Ten Denied DRGs, Hospital Payment Monitoring Program. http://providers.ipro.org/index/hpmp.

UVA. 2008. University of Virginia (UVA) Medical Center Reduces Coding Errors with Six Sigma. Report On Medicare Compliance. http://healthcare.isixsigma.com/library/content/c030501a.asp.

Chapter 10
Collecting, Analyzing, and Reporting on Program Data

Chapter 9 discussed the collection of key metrics for the query process. These metrics include the record review rate, query rate, physician response rate, and query agreement (or validation) rate. These are the core operational measures that every organization must collect to ensure a smooth and continuous process. However, there are also additional measures that can be collected for strategic and management purposes, as well as for reviewing and analyzing the data for key metrics. As with all other program design elements, it is essential that an organization develop program data reporting means that are specific to its needs. In the author's experience, no two programs use exactly the same program data reporting. While the key metrics for querying are always used as the base data, every program has some specific nuances around the other data it collects and reviews and how it uses this data. Examples of data from different programs are provided in this chapter.

Essential Data Elements

The core key metric table from chapter 9 is provided again in table 10.1 as a review of the key data elements that should form the basis for data analysis for every CDI program. While the data elements of record review rate, query rate, response rate, and validation rate are the same, the targets set for each metric should be organization-specific (Tangen 2003). They should also be targets that are both achievable and challenging.

Figure 10.1 depicts the process and timing for collection of each of the key metrics. Both the concurrent and retrospective review and query process are represented in the figure. Physician response, if obtained, occurs after review and query.

Additional Ways to Analyze Core Key Metrics

It is important to report on and analyze the CDI core key metrics in the aggregate. However, it is also helpful to generate reports that present the data in different manners. For example, the record review rate in table 10.1 was 75 percent overall. It may be helpful to report on the record review rate by CDI specialist, nursing unit, or service. Looking at the review rate by CDI specialist can identify productivity problems by individual. Review rate by nursing unit or service could identify if there are problems obtaining the patient records in certain units. If so, the units or services could be contacted and appropriate problem-solving activities can follow. This analysis is only helpful for organizations with hard-copy health records because those with electronic health records should

Table 10.1   Sample clinical documentation key measures

Key Metric	Quarter 1	Target*	% Achievement
Concurrent: Record review rate	75%	90%	83%
Concurrent: Physician **query** rate	40%	40%	100%
Physician **response** rate	50%	75%	67%
Physician **validation** rate	70%	80%	88%
Retrospective: Physician **query** rate	5%	15%	33%
Physician **response** rate	100%	60%	60%
Physician **validation** rate	65%	85%	76%

*Note: The targets noted were created specifically by the healthcare organization using its own assessment data. All targets should be organization-specific and be validated on at least an annual basis.

Figure 10.1   Collection of operational core CDI key metrics

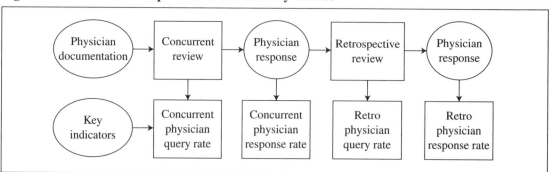

usually not have access problems. Access problems with an EHR indicate either a shortage of terminals or a wait time for data transfer or streaming that should be addressed by the information technology (IT) department.

Table 10.2 shows an example of the CDI core key metrics broken down by CDI specialist. The preliminary data analysis of this table shows that reviewers B, C, and E all appear to be producing results that are consistent with the target rates for the organization. Reviewers A, D, and F have produced some outcomes that need to be investigated further. For example, reviewer A is reviewing many more records than the others, but the query rate is much lower. This may represent rushed reviews. However, when these data elements are viewed in light of the agreement rate of 98 percent, it may actually represent more careful reviews and interactions with the physicians. The agreement rate of 98 percent may also represent leading queries or overly aggressive interactions with the physicians. In any case, individual metrics that are significantly different from the targets and the rest of the group, especially for more than a one-month period, need to be investigated through discussion, review of the queries, possibly concurrent observation of the reviewer and follow-up education to correct any gaps in skill or knowledge.

Reviewer D has the opposite problem of reviewer A. Reviewer D's review rate is much lower at 60 percent. But, the query rate is much higher at 50 percent. This may simply represent a productivity issue that, if corrected, would result in a query rate consistent with the targets. The agreement rate of 95 percent is also a concern and needs to be investigated. Finally, reviewer F's metrics are consistent with the exception of the agreement rate. At 29 percent, the concern is the validity of the queries reviewer F is generating, and the metric may represent a gap in skills that needs to be corrected (UVA 2008).

Table 10.2   CDI core key metrics for concurrent queries by CDI specialist

CDI Specialist	Concurrent Review Rate	Concurrent Query Rate	Concurrent Response Rate	Concurrent Agreement Rate
A	97%	20%	67%	98%
B	80%	30%	65%	69%
C	82%	33%	68%	70%
D	60%	50%	90%	95%
E	80%	28%	63%	72%
F	85%	29%	65%	29%

Table 10.3   CDI core key metrics for concurrent queries by service

Service	Concurrent Query Rate	Concurrent Response Rate	Concurrent Agreement Rate
Internal medicine	35%	68%	65%
Cardiology	25%	80%	30%
Neurology	10%	75%	60%
Gastroenterology	35%	70%	75%
General surgery	40%	50%	60%
Orthopedic surgery	55%	35%	30%
Cardiac surgery	30%	62%	70%
Urology	36%	78%	70%
OB/GYN	25%	70%	80%

Table 10.3 contains the core key metrics by specialty for concurrent queries only. If necessary, this information can be further broken down by individual physicians to identify who may need follow-up training. The data on this table show a problem with general surgery and orthopedic surgery. For the orthopedic service, the query rate at 55 percent is much higher than the target of 33 percent. Furthermore, the response rates for both services are lower than the targets. And, the orthopedic surgery agreement rate is significantly lower than the target rate of 75 percent. The initial follow-up to this should be both a review of a sampling of these records and discussion with the chiefs of each service, followed by the appropriate follow-up education or discussions to obtain support from the physicians who respond to the queries.

The primary purpose of collecting and reviewing core key metrics is to identify any gaps in knowledge or skills and take the appropriate corrective action. Even when the key metrics are consistent with target rates, records should be reviewed and audits should occur to validate the reviews and the target rates. These activities are discussed in more detail in chapter 11 on program compliance.

Collection and Analysis of Additional Operational Data Elements

Most programs collect operational key metrics in addition to the core metrics. These metrics are often determined as the program matures and the management team is able to identify additional areas of interest or concern. Some, however, are metrics that are and should be reviewed from the inception of the program. Some of the key metrics that should be reviewed regularly include the reason for the query, the types of secondary diagnoses added on review, and the types of principal diagnosis changes that were made. These metrics can only be reviewed if the appropriate data is collected at the time of the CDI specialist's review.

The reason for query is often focused on the type of documentation that prompted the query. For example, common ways to categorize a reason for query include:

- Abnormal laboratory tests not addressed

- Abnormal radiology tests

- Medication ordered without a supporting diagnosis

- Conflicting documentation between the attending physician and the consultant

This type of information is helpful to collect because it can be used to focus follow-up education. For example, if the data tells us that 52 percent of all queries were due to abnormal laboratory tests not addressed by the physician, follow-up communication and education can be designed appropriately.

The type of impact produced by the physician's response can also be helpful to analyze. For example, in most cases, additional documentation from the physician is likely to result in either an additional diagnosis added, a different principal diagnosis being supported, a more refined diagnosis (either principal or secondary), or an additional or more specific procedure (IPRO 2005a; IPRO 2005b). If trends of certain diagnoses or procedures can be identified over time, this information can be used to design follow-up education targeted at specific physicians, services, or the entire medical staff if the documentation problem appears to be a global one.

Tables 10.4 and 10.5 are examples of reports that show, over time, the types of diagnoses added and principal diagnosis changes, as a result of query responses. Table 10.4 shows that the most significant changes in principal diagnosis were due to sepsis. This information should be used to create follow-up training specific to documentation for sepsis and related conditions such as that discussed in chapter 9.

Table 10.5 shows the diagnoses most commonly added to patient records as a result of physician responses to queries. In this case, anemia, electrolyte imbalance, and heart arrhythmias were the top three most common conditions. This information, analyzed in conjunction with metrics about the reason for query or the location of documentation supporting a query can be used to design brief, focused follow-up education. For example, if the arrhythmias were added because physicians were not documenting diagnoses from the electrocardiogram (EKG) into the progress notes, then copies of EKGs from those records can be used during follow-up education to demonstrate to physicians that cardiologists' documentation (the nontreating physician) cannot be relied upon in the record to translate information into coded data (CMS 2006a; CMS 2006b; MedPAC 2006).

Table 10.4   Principal diagnosis metrics from CDI query responses

Changed to this principal diagnosis	# Times
Sepsis (from bacteremia)	7
Acute congestive heart failure (from CHF NOS)	6
Respiratory failure (from other respiratory diagnoses)	3

Table 10.5   Secondary diagnosis key metrics from CDI query responses

Diagnosis added after query	# Times added
Anemia NOS	29
Electrolyte imbalance (hypo or hypernatremia, hypo or hyperkalemia, hypo or hypercalcemia)	25
Arrhythmias (atrial fibrillation, bradycardia, tachycardia,ventricular tachycardia)	25
Intravenous drug abuse	17
Urinary tract infection	15
Pneumonia	15
Hypertension	15
Reflux esophagitis	12
Obesity	11
Loss of consciousness	11
Chronic renal failure	11
Acute renal failure	11
Tobacco abuse	10
Hypercholesterolemia	10
Dehydration	10
Blood loss anemia	10
CHF	9
Atelectasis	9
Thrombocytopenia	7
Malnourished	7
Hypotension	7

Collection and Analysis of Strategic Data Elements

Up to this point, the data elements that have been discussed are primarily used to steer program operations. However, the executive team can also use program data to make strategic decisions. In fact, to the extent that the executive team relies upon data produced by the CDI program, and that data shows positive impact to the organization, the opportunity exists to continue to expand the clinical documentation function in the organization. There are four key areas in which the executive team has an interest in reviewing data. These areas all impact, to some degree, the strategic key metrics of quality, profitability, physician satisfaction, and patient satisfaction. It may be necessary for the CDI team to demonstrate these relationships, but as demonstrated in the following sections, a clear relationship can be found between strategic decision making and the data obtained from a CDI program.

Case Mix Index

Case mix index (CMI), which is the average DRG relative weight for inpatient cases, is an indicator of average reimbursement per patient (MedPAC 2006). For example, if a hospital's CMI is 1.2 and the blended rate is $6,000, then average reimbursement is $7,200. If CMI increases, the average reimbursement increases. If CMI decreases, the average reimbursement decreases. Because of the relationship between revenue, profit and CMI, healthcare managers have a strong interest in tracking CMI. They also have a strong interest in understanding any activity that impacts their organization's CMI, including the organization's clinical documentation practices. In particular, if documentation practices were not of high quality prior to implementation of the program, which would have been identified during the assessment, it is possible that improved documentation quality will have a positive impact on CMI.

Documentation and coding can impact CMI. When documentation impacts CMI, it is called CDI case mix change. However, it is important that the senior executives in the organization are tracking other indicators of case mix change as well. Significant CMI change can occur when the types of patients admitted to the hospital change (Rosko and Chilingerian 1999). This is known as real patient case mix change. The following components can impact the CMI:

- Seasonal variations

- Medical and surgical mix

- Physician staffing changes

- Coding competency

- Severity of illnesses among the patient population

The two types of CMI change, real patient mix change and documentation CMI change are described in more detail below.

Real Patient Mix Change

Real patient mix change is a change in case mix index that occurs as a result of different types of patients being admitted and treated at the hospital in a given time period as compared to a prior time period. For example, during the month of November, a hospital discharged 100 patients with 25 being patients who received a surgical procedure. During November, the CMI was 2.0. Then, in December, 100 patients were discharged, but only 10 patients received a surgical procedure, and the remaining patients were medical patients. The CMI was 1.3. The change in CMI from November to December in this case was due to a real patient mix change caused by less demand for surgery. This type of CMI change can not be improved by documentation improvement activities. It is important for executives to understand when they have had a CMI change, either increase or decrease, what part of the change, if any, was due to real patient mix change, and not CDI activities.

CDI Case Mix Change

CDI case mix change is a change in case mix index that occurs as a result of a change in documentation practices. For example, in the month of November, a hospital's complication and comorbidity (CC) capture rate was 85 percent and the CMI was 2.0. Then, in the month of December, CC capture rate fell to 72 percent and the CMI was 1.5. When December cases without a CC were reviewed retrospectively (after the time period for resubmission), it was identified that 20 percent of these cases were cases where the physician did not document the clinical significance (diagnosis) for abnormal test results. This same review identified that during the month of November, physicians had been documenting the reason and diagnosis for abnormal test results. The change in CMI from

November to December is due to documentation practices. And, the research behind it can be traced to link CMI with those documentation practices. This is an example of where the CDI program can impact the hospital's CMI.

It is helpful to illustrate changes in CMI with graphs. In general, all graphic illustrations shared throughout an organization should be accompanied by an explanation of the significance of the data illustrated on the graph. This practice avoids confusion and misinterpretation.

An example of a clear, simple graph appears in figure 10.2. The explanation accompanying the graph can read:

> This graph shows a decrease in surgical mix from a mean of 34 percent in 2004 to 25 percent in 2005.

Because surgery cases are valued by the DRG system at approximately 2.25 times medical cases, this drop in surgical mix has had a significant impact on the hospital's overall case mix. This demonstrates a real patient mix change. The best possible documentation could not make up for a real change in patient mix. It is imperative that senior executives in the organization understand this concept and can differentiate between what documentation can legitimately impact and what it cannot impact. CDI program managers can ensure these types of concepts are understood throughout the organization by sharing this kind of information, if it is not already collected and analyzed.

The graph in figure 10.3 is used to link the change in medical and surgical mix to the change in case mix index. The following explanation can accompany this graph:

> The Medicare CMI has shown a steady downward trend since June. This could be, in large part, due to the decline in the number of surgical cases relative to medical cases. With the exception of Blue Cross payers, all payers have shown a declining CMI since April.

Figure 10.2   Medical and surgical cases by month: 2004 to 2005 monthly comparison

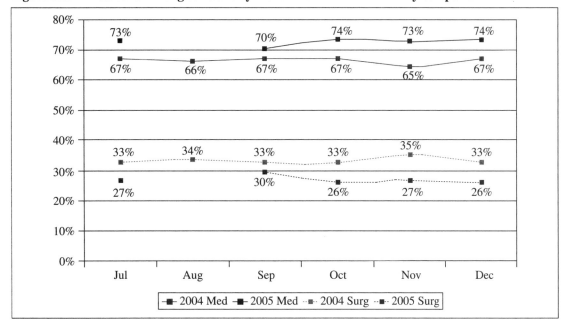

Figure 10.3   Hospital-wide CMI by month

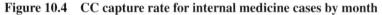

Figure 10.4   CC capture rate for internal medicine cases by month

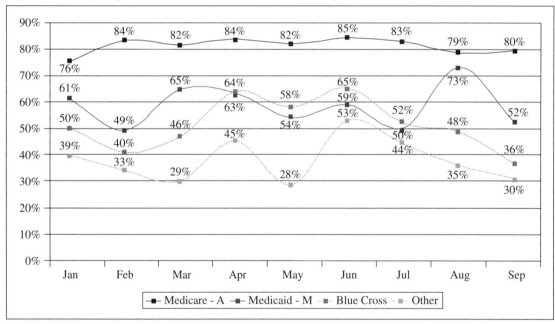

In addition to overall CMI, most hospital administrators track CMI by service and CC capture rate. Figures 10.4 and 10.5 are graphs that illustrate the comparison of CMI by service and CC capture rate for the internal medicine service over time. To the extent that an increase (or decrease) in CMI or CC capture rate is not accompanied by a real patient mix change, clinical documentation changes (better or worse) may be responsible for all or part of the CMI and CC capture rate changes.

Figure 10.5   Case mix index (CMI) for internal medicine cases by month

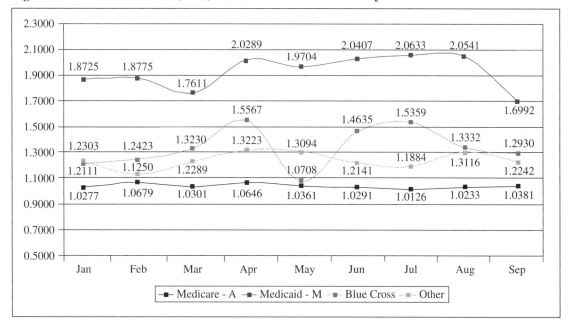

Quality Indicators and Severity of Illness Analysis

Most quality reporting systems, including Medicare quality indicators and Health-Grades, use the APR severity DRGs to calculate quality ratings. The APR system uses a four-level severity rating system for all cases (Averill et al. 2003). Severity level 1 is the lowest severity rating and severity level 4 is the highest severity rating. Although the specific methodologies by private organizations like HealthGrades are not known, in general, hospitals can count on better quality ratings if the majority of their inpatients are grouped into higher severity levels. Hospitals with fewer severity level 1 cases (usually less than 20 percent) are more likely to fare better in the ratings than a peer with 30 percent of its inpatient cases grouped into severity level 1. Some of this makes basic intuitive sense. Why would an acute care hospital, whose focus is treating acute, severely ill patients, have any sizable number of severity level 1 patients? An argument could be made that no inpatient cases should ever be grouped into severity level 1, which is a mild level of severity. From a medical necessity perspective, the question can be asked whether severity level 1 patients need inpatient care at all.

Ultimately, the higher the quality of the clinical documentation in a patient record, the more likely that a hospital's severity levels will be accurate. Many hospitals that implement clinical documentation programs see an initial increase in severity levels. Figure 10.6 is an example of pre- and post-CDI severity level changes. The graph shows that over time the hospital's percentage of severity level 1 cases decreased from a high of 32 percent to a low of 16 percent. In addition, severity level 4 cases increased from a low of 6 percent to a high of 16 percent. Severity level 2 cases showed little change and severity level 3 cases showed some increase. After analysis, it was clear that higher quality clinical documentation was the primary contributor to these severity level changes. Therefore, by tracking APR severity levels, an organization can predict changes in how they are represented to the public in quality ratings and healthcare report cards.

Figure 10.6   Severity level changes over time

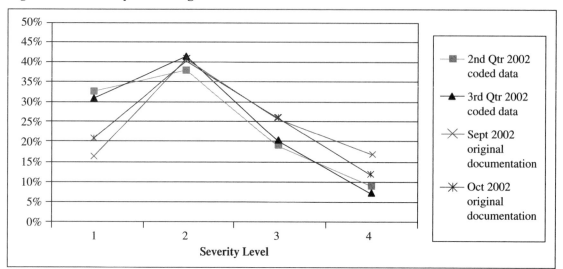

Figure 10.7.   Severity levels by physician

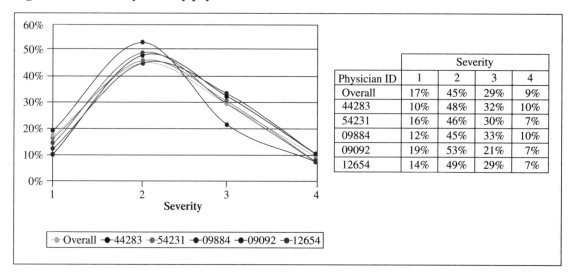

	Severity			
Physician ID	1	2	3	4
Overall	17%	45%	29%	9%
44283	10%	48%	32%	10%
54231	16%	46%	30%	7%
09884	12%	45%	33%	10%
09092	19%	53%	21%	7%
12654	14%	49%	29%	7%

Hospitals can also track inpatient severity level differences by physician. This analysis can help determine if there is a particular physician or group of physicians who are contributing to the hospital's low levels of severity through documentation or possibly admitting patients who may not meet the criteria for medical necessity for an acute care admission. Figure 10.7 shows an example of severity level tracking by physician. The table next to the graph shows that physician 09092 has a significantly lower average patient severity than the other physicians. This information can likely be traced back to some problems with the physician's clinical documentation practices.

Physician Response Rate

Physician response rate is one of the core key metrics discussed at the beginning of the chapter. It is included here in the section on strategy because physician response rate can be evidence of physician-hospital alignment or lack thereof. Senior executives in the hospital should track the physician response rate for this reason. In particular, knowing which physicians may be consistently unresponsive will give the organization's leadership some idea about where they may need to be working on some relationship building. Alternatively, for those physicians who are consistent responders, the hospital should be showing its appreciation in an appropriate and regular way to these physicians.

Patient Satisfaction

Patient satisfaction is a new consideration in its relationship to clinical documentation. One hypothesis is that because patients are more likely to request and review their health records today than they were a decade ago, the documentation in their record may impact their level of satisfaction with the hospital's services overall. This can be measured in an indirect way through patient satisfaction surveys whenever a patient requests a health record. But mostly, at this point, patient satisfaction related to health information is an indirect strategic measure. Patients have the right to request changes to the information in their health records as a result of HIPAA, and they are more likely to pay close attention to that information (HIPAA 1996). Today, it is most helpful for physicians to consider the role of the patient regarding documented health information, which the patient owns.

Review of Sample CDI Dashboard

Every organization will need to design its own dashboard of CDI metrics. A performance dashboard is a tool that provides timely and relevant information so processes can be measured and managed. Table 10.6 is an example of a CDI dashboard that contains both strategic and operational metrics. The core metrics of response and query rate are captured here. In addition, monthly severity levels are tracked and analyzed. In this particular organization much time was spent determining which inpatient cases were eligible for CDI review, based on length-of-stay criteria. To ensure that everyone in the organization had the same idea about which cases were eligible for review, this information was included with the metrics collected monthly. HIM querying and documentation compliance were also concerns, and they were tracked as well.

Conclusion

There is an enormous amount of information that is generated through a CDI program. Every organization must plan for how that information will be captured, reported, and analyzed. Key metrics, along with their targets, can be used to analyze current performance and implement continuous improvements to the program. In addition, data can be analyzed not only organization wide, but also by service, physician, and CDI specialist. This detailed data reporting can help identify gaps in knowledge and skill sets of specific individuals who can then be involved in focused follow-up training to close the gaps.

Table 10.6   Sample CDI dashboard with strategic and operational metrics

		January	February	March	April	YTD 06
Concurrent Queries						
	# Queries placed	414	440	676	567	4,461
	Response rate *(Target = 90%)*	31%	32%	28%	40%	36%
Concurrent Reviews						
	# Patient reviews completed	794	826	893	864	7,946
	# Patients eligible for CDI review	1,407	1,405	1,476	1,356	14,024
	% of eligible patients reviewed *(Target = 85%)*	56%	59%	61%	64%	57%
	# 1-day LOS reviewed	94	78	70	77	834
	% Patient reviews with 1 or more queries	52%	53%	76%	66%	56%
	% CDI reviews with severity assigned	98%	98%	96%	93%	78%
Retrospective Queries by HIM						
	# Queries placed	9	18	24	88	172
	Response rate	22%	44%	21%	8%	18%
Process Flow						
	# CDI reviews accessed in CDI system by HIM	594	583	595	693	4,422
Documentation Compliance						
	Charts missing documentation at time of coding	651	572	899	886	5,463
Quarterly Change in Severity Level						
Level 1	Level 1 *(Target = <18%)*	18%	18%	15%	14%	
Level 2	Level 2	42%	42%	42%	40%	
Level 3	Level 3	28%	27%	28%	31%	
Level 4	Level 4	14%	13%	14%	15%	

References

42 CFR 3. 2007. Medicare Conditions of Participation.

Averill, R. F., G. Norbert., J. S. Hughes, et al. 2003. *All Patient Refined Diagnosis-Related Groups, Definitions Manual, Version 20.0, Volumes 1, 2, and 3*. Wallingford, CT: 3M Health Information Systems.

Centers for Medicare and Medicaid Services (CMS) and the National Center for Health Statistics (NCHS). 2006a. ICD-9-CM Official Guidelines for Coding and Reporting. www.cdc.gov/nchs/datawh/ftpserv/ftpicd9/ftpicd9.htm.

Centers for Medicare and Medicaid Services (CMS) and the National Center for Health Statistics (NCHS). 2006b. ICD-9-CM Official Guidelines for Coding and Reporting—Supplement. http://www.cdc.gov/nchs/data/icd9/POAguideSep06.pdf.

IPRO. 2005a. Coding for Quality: Documentation tips for the Top Seven DRGs Revised 2005, Hospital Payment Monitoring Program. http://providers.ipro.org/index/hpmp.

IPRO. 2005b. Coding for Quality: Documentation tips for the Top Ten Denied DRGs, Hospital Payment Monitoring Program. http://providers.ipro.org/index/hpmp.

MedPAC. 2006. Payment Basic: Hospital Acute Inpatient Services Payment System. http:www.medpac.gov/publications/other-reports/Sept06_MedPAC_Payment-Basics_hospital.pdf.

Rosko, M. D. and J. A. Chilingerian. 1999. Estimating hospital inefficiency: Does case mix matter? *Journal of Medical Systems*. 23(1):57–71.

Tangen, S. 2003. An overview of frequently used performance measures. *Journal of Work Study*. 52(7):347–354.

UVA. 2008. University of Virginia (UVA) Medical Center Reduces Coding Errors with Six Sigma. Report On Medicare Compliance. http://healthcare.isixsigma.com/library/ content/c030501a.asp.

Chapter 11
Ensuring CDI Program Compliance

Regulatory compliance is a concern for every healthcare organization. In particular any activities that impact the coding and billing process are scrutinized by CMS and HHS' Office of the Inspector General in their annual work plans for healthcare organizations. Since clinical documentation is translated by coding professionals into the diagnostic and procedural codes that are the basis for billing, it has the potential to be closely monitored by regulatory agencies. Additionally, compliance investigations that involve over-billing to the federal government can result in treble damages and fines of up to $10,000 per occurrence, as well as the possibility of exclusion from the Medicare program, not to mention significant legal and consulting fees. Therefore, all healthcare organizations should manage their operations to ensure compliance (HHS 1999; HHS 1998). This chapter addresses the basic components of a compliance program as they relate to clinical documentation practices and discusses in detail the activities of monitoring, auditing, and follow-up education.

Overview of Compliance

An organizational compliance program is developed under the direction of the organization's compliance officer, and it applies to all operations throughout the organization. As discussed in previous chapters, an organization's compliance officer should be involved in the oversight committee for CDI and should be part of the senior management team that works to build physician support for the program. The CDI function is included, to some degree, in every organization's compliance plan. The CDI function is also likely to be included in some level of annual auditing that is managed by the compliance department. Day-to-day monitoring, however, is the responsibility of the CDI department. It is a responsibility, under an organization's compliance plan, to document the monitoring process and report the results to the compliance officer on a regular basis. Other interactions between operational units of the organization and the compliance team will vary depending on the organization and the compliance department. The CDI program manager should check in with the compliance officer to make sure that he or she has provided the department with the information it needs and to ensure that any responsibilities the CDI program has are clear to the compliance function in terms of regular reporting.

The best way for every operation within an organization to manage itself is to design its day-to-day processes that include at the operational level, the four components of a compliance plan. These components are:

1. Policy and procedure development

2. Program monitoring

3. Auditing

4. Follow-up education (HHS 1999; HHS 1998)

Ideally, the CDI program should have documentation and processes in place that address each of these areas. Should there ever be an external or internal inquiry about possible compliance violations of the program, not only would the data from the compliance department be available, but the CDI program's operational documentation from these four areas would be available as well.

Earlier chapters of the book discussed program policies and procedure development. Program monitoring, auditing, and follow-up education are activities that continue on an ongoing basis. There are however, three key components that should be in place for every CDI program to ensure compliance from the outset.

Three Key Components of a Compliant CDI Program

The three key components of a compliant CDI program that should be in place as early in the program implementation as possible include:

1. Documented, mandatory physician education

2. Detailed query documentation

3. CDI policies and procedures with annual sign-off from all program staff

These activities have significant synergy and interface directly with the compliance department's activities. First, documented, mandatory physician education should be the initial step in every CDI program. Clinical documentation should be implemented through the medical staff, not around them. They are the authors of the documentation. Implementing a CDI program without first informing the physicians about their rights and responsibilities in the CDI process could present problems in the future. Comprehensive training programs attended by all physicians, preferably with follow-up testing, is the best process to follow. Post-education testing, also discussed with follow-up education, is excellent evidence for compliance purposes. Test results serve as evidence of what the trainee knew (and did not know). In the course of a compliance investigation, follow-up education and test results can be used, for example, to support the fact that a problem was identified by the organization and addressed through these vehicles.

Second, every program should keep detailed query data. There should be documented evidence of all queries that were asked, the clinical documentation or information in the record supporting the query, to whom it was asked, and the response to the query. This documentation should even accompany every verbal query. For verbal queries, the CDI specialist may need to document the query and the response in the program database. But, in no event should a query be asked and answered without documented evidence that it occurred. There are some concerns by CMS and the QIOs surrounding verbal queries. This can be managed by hospitals' development of a practice to document all query interactions.

Detailed query documentation can also be used to protect the hospital against any possible claims from physicians that they were asked leading queries or they felt they were being forced into documenting in a certain way. Query documentation coupled with mandatory training programs where physicians are trained in the seven criteria for high-quality clinical documentation as well as their rights and responsibilities in their own clinical documentation is some of the strongest support an organization can have for a compliant CDI process. Coupling query documentation and training with post-training tests successfully completed by all physicians ensures a solid compliance program (HHS 1999; Russo and Fitzgerald 2008).

Lastly, it is important to develop and continuously update policies and procedures for the CDI program. Moreover, it is just as important to ensure that staff members are familiar with the policies and procedures that impact them. Training sessions can be developed to review key policies and procedures with staff. In these cases, testing staff members on the content of the training is the best evidence that they know how to apply the policies. Alternately, staff members can read the policies and procedures independently, but they should also be tested on content and sign off on the fact that they have read the policies and procedures and agree to abide by them.

Monitoring the CDI Program

All CDI staff members need to have their work reviewed and monitored on an ongoing basis to ensure quality. The CDI program manager, or consulting team if an outside firm is used for implementation, should begin this process in the form of shadowing during implementation. If a consulting firm is managing the implementation process, the responsibility for ongoing monitoring should be transitioned to the internal CDI program manager as early in the follow-up visit process as possible. Every organization will develop its own methodology for conducting regular monitoring. At a minimum, the CDI core key metrics can be used to determine if there are any areas of concern that need to be focused on in the current reviews. Some suggestions for creating a regular monitoring process follow.

Reviews should be conducted concurrently, after the CDI specialist has reviewed records on the unit. This will provide the best opportunity to provide feedback based upon the exact content of the record at the time the CDI specialist reviewed it. Targets for overall proficiency of queries should be in the 90 to 95 percent range. The quality reviews should measure the same areas that the program database measures: query rates, reason for query, and location of documentation supporting the query. Productivity should be checked, but also the query rate, response rate, and agreement rate should be reviewed. Each of these rates plays an important role in identifying the performance level of the CDI specialist. As was noted in chapter 9, if there is a low agreement rate (more than 10 percentage points below the target), it may indicate the CDI specialist is asking inappropriate queries.

During a CDI quality review, the following elements should be tracked and monitored:

- Validity of queries generated
- Validity of working DRG assignment
- Validity of CDI specialist's DRG assignment
- Missed query opportunity

Table 11.1 shows a form used for concurrent CDI reviews. The form focuses on validating queries or missed query opportunities. Data elements can be modified to fit the specific needs of an organization. Ideally, the data elements would be entered directly into a program's database for analysis and reporting. Monitoring data should be collected at least monthly and reviewed at least quarterly. However, some organizations may want to collect and review data weekly and monthly. It is important to review and analyze results on a regular basis so that any gaps in skills or knowledge identified by the review can be corrected through education or program modifications.

Every program should include regular observation of the query process. For example, a CDI program manager may select one day a month to visit the units and observe verbal queries posed directly to physicians by the CDI specialists. The CDI program manager may also listen to discussions between physicians and the CDI specialists about previous queries. During the observation, the CDI program manager should document the interaction between the CDI specialist and the physician. In particular, the manager should note whether the query was:

1. Supported by clinical evidence and what the evidence was

2. Asked in a nonleading manner

3. Responded to by the physician through appropriate documentation in the patient record

The organization can design a simple form to record this information. The form should allow the CDI program manager to assess whether the interaction was leading, the demeanor of the physician, the outcome of the discussion, and any other comments. A copy of the form should be filed with other program data, and a copy should be given to the CDI specialist with the appropriate feedback. The CDI program manager should schedule observations so that all CDI specialists can be assessed on their interaction with physicians at least twice a year.

Auditing the CDI Program

A comprehensive review of all query opportunities should be conducted retrospectively at least once a year. This audit can be performed internally, however, the organization will likely benefit from bringing in an outside firm to perform the annual audit. Primary focus of the CDI audit is to validate that the program is operating compliantly

Table 11.1   Sample CDI monitoring form

MR#/ Name	Admit Date	Working DRG	Agree? Y/N	If no, Audit DRG	CDS DRG	Agree? Y/N	If no, Audit DRG	Concurrent Query Type	Agree? Y/N	If no, Audit query	Missed Query Opportunities
99999	2/1/06	90	Y		89	Y		Dehydration	Y		
99998	2/3/06	320	Y		320	Y		None	N		Abn Labs
Totals											

and achieving program goals. The quality component assesses whether the reviews generated appropriate queries, whether the query forms were completed accurately, and whether the physician's documentation in response to a query was appropriate. Issues in any of these areas should be identified in the audit, reported on, and followed up with education or changes in the program process. Focused follow-up education is the key to keeping a CDI program in compliance.

Sample Selection

The sample is selected from the population, which is defined as all records that were concurrently reviewed for CDI purposes, regardless of whether a query was asked. In general, a valid review requires a minimum of 30 cases in the sample (Wang et al. 1995, 53). There are many other decisions to be made regarding the sample selection process. One of the most important considerations is that the sample-selection decisions made for the first review must remain constant in all future reviews if results are to be compared among different reviews. Since comparison of audit results is preferred and usually helpful, it is important to make good initial decisions about sample selection (and even the review and data collection process). The more carefully thought out the initial decisions are, the greater is the chance that the program will have useful historical data for comparison over time. Sample-selection decisions should be carefully documented so the methodology can be reproduced in the future.

Whether the review will select records for concurrent or retrospective review must also be determined. Each method has its own pros and cons and every organization has different needs. The decisions should be based on each organization's specific needs and capabilities. It is both easier to obtain a random sample and more efficient to audit using a retrospective review. A retrospective documentation review minimizes the issue of bias that may exist when reviewers know they are being audited (as they do during a concurrent audit). However, with a retrospective audit, it is more difficult to recreate the actual situation that existed at the time the CDI specialist was reviewing the patient record. One commonly-used option consists of auditing the majority of records retrospectively and then including 10 to 20 cases concurrently. The cases need to be reported on differently, but the process often reveals issues in the concurrent practice that would not have been uncovered during a retrospective review.

The number of records for review also must be determined. As noted initially, 30 is the minimum. The size of the organization may require that more records be reviewed to obtain a representative sample. For outpatient cases, 100 or more cases may be needed to obtain a representative sampling. For inpatient cases, one methodology to use is the number of beds in the hospital involved in the CDI process. For example, a hospital has 150 beds. Obstetrics and newborn, which represent 20 beds, are currently excluded from the program. Furthermore, about 10 percent of hospital admissions are one-day stays, which represents 15 beds. The total beds involved in the program then are 115 (150 − (20 + 15) = 115). Auditing 25 percent of bed size would mean a review of 30 records. However, the organization may want to audit 50 percent, which would be 60 records. There is no magic number in this process. What is important is that the decision can be maintained for future audits.

Random sampling versus focused sampling is another issue to be addressed. It is almost impossible to select a truly random sample in a concurrent CDI review because of the nature of the review process. For a retrospective review, cases can be selected randomly. However, the compliance department may have a concern about random reviews based on the fact that a problem that impacts reimbursement may trigger a pay-back process. When this is the case, a convenience sampling may be preferred. Convenience sampling can be done by pulling the last 30 discharges that had a concurrent CDI review, or by pulling 10 discharges from three different time periods in the last quarter to ensure seasonality representation. Essentially, a convenience sample is just what the word states: selecting cases that are convenient to retrieve. When this methodology is used, as long as the same methodology used in the future, results of different audits can be compared (Babbie 1999).

Record Review

The record review process should be conducted by qualified individuals who are not involved in the day-to-day operations of the CDI program. The methodology for review should be consistent among all reviewers and for each audit conducted. For example, at the time of review, the record should be in as close as possible a condition to the way it was when the CDI specialist reviewed it. For a retrospective review, this can be particularly challenging. However, it is helpful to document how the auditors will view the record. For instance, for all retrospective reviews, it is important that the auditor not refer to the discharge summary or any documentation that was not available to the CDI specialist at the time of the concurrent review.

Data Collection and Analysis

It is also important to determine what data elements will be collected by the reviewer and how they will be collected. Some data elements to consider include:

1. The CDI reviewer's name

2. Whether a query was asked (yes or no)

3. If a query was asked:

   —Does the auditor agree with it?

   —Where was the location of the documentation supporting the query?

   —What type of documentation and coding changes resulted from the query (IPRO 2005a; IPRO 2005b; CMS 2006a; CMS 2006b)?

4. If a query was not asked:

   —Was there a lost query opportunity? If yes, what was it?

   —Can a retrospective query be asked at this time?

5. If the physician responded

6. If the physician did not respond

7. DRG assignment

8. Severity assignment

Figure 11.1 presents an example of a data collection form that can used or modified for use in a clinical documentation audit. One audit form would be completed for each record reviewed. The form can also be used to collect information about retrospective queries, if desired.

Figure 11.1.   Sample data collection form

Medical Record			
Account Number #:		Coder ID:	
APR-DRG/SOI Assignment			
CDS Name	**Admit Date**	**CDS Review Date**	**Working APR-DRG/SOI**
CDS (target) Severity DRG/SOI	Coder DRG/APR-DRG/SOI	Final DRG/ APR-DRG/SOI	Coder Relative Weight Variance (coder & final)
Concurrent Query Response Verification			
Concurrent Query	**Recorded Response**	**Audited Response**	**If "y" condition coded?**
	Y N NR A	Y N NR A	Y N
	Y N NR A	Y N NR A	Y N
	Y N NR A	Y N NR A	Y N
	Y N NR A	Y N NR A	Y N
	Y N NR A	Y N NR A	Y N
	Y N NR A	Y N NR A	Y N
	Y N NR A	Y N NR A	Y N

"N" "NR" or "A" Retrospective Queries				
Concurrent Query	**Response**	**Condition Documented in Record (not coded)**	**Impacting Query**	**Re-Queried?**
	N NR A	Y N	Y N	Y N
	N NR A	Y N	Y N	Y N
	N NR A	Y N	Y N	Y N
	N NR A	Y N	Y N	Y N
	N NR A	Y N	Y N	Y N
	N NR A	Y N	Y N	Y N
	N NR A	Y N	Y N	Y N

Missed Coder or CDS Query Impact		
Missed Query	**APR-DRG Impact**	**Relative Weight Impact**

Developing a Corrective Action Plan

Most audits should identify some issues, either operational or compliance, in the CDI process, even if they are minor issues. Some organizations use an issue rating system for every issue identified on an audit. The system may be from 1 through 5 with a level 1 issue being minor and only operational in nature and a level 5 being significant or potentially significant and compliance in nature. The organization needs to develop a corrective action plan for any issues identified. The correction action plan should include individual communications, training, testing, and operational changes that will be made. The plan should include dates for completion and a checklist that needs to be completed and filed with program documentation when all of the corrective actions have been completed.

Reporting on Results

Every audit should be summarized in a report. The design of the the report format should be specific to the needs of the organization, as should how and to whom the audit results will be presented. For example, will the results be presented at a CDI committee meeting? Will copies of the results be forwarded to the compliance department in every case or only when the review has identified compliance concerns? If possible, the reports should be designed to enable easy comparison of results over time. The first page of the report can contain an executive summary that lists the basic data findings. For each audit, the report can include the findings from the previous two reviews to show changes over time.

Follow-up Education and Testing

The goal of any compliance review is to determine whether query generation and physician responses to the queries are being performed compliantly. If either activity is determined to be lacking in compliance, then a corrective action plan must be developed. The most common and generally most useful corrective action plan uses focused follow-up education. Details around ensuring attendance at educational programs by physicians and designing program content have been addressed in earlier chapters. This chapter will concentrate on the design and use of post-education testing as a tool for compliance.

Focused follow-up education should be designed to address every issue identified as the result of an audit or during monitoring. All issues should be clearly documented in the audit or monitoring report. The general plan for educational follow-up to correct these issues should also be included in the report. Organizations should create and maintain detailed documentation for every training program. The content of the program, attendance at the sessions, and results of any post-training tests should be maintained by the CDI program manager. Ideally, the documentation should be electronic and any hard copy documents should be imaged into the electronic filing system. Every training program should include the following components:

1. Objectives: The objectives to be achieved through the training should be clearly stated and provided to all attendees as part of the program materials. If the organization is to provide continuing education credits, most professional associations require a list of educational objectives. These objectives should be used to create the content of the program. They should also be used to design any post-training tests.

2. Training method: The CAMP Method should be used for optimal outcomes. The CAMP Method was reviewed previously as the best method for educating adults. Use of this method not only improves skills, it also increases the sustainability of the training. See chapter 7 for an overview of the four components of the CAMP method and how to incorporate them into the training program (Russo and Fitzgerald 2008).

3. The right trainers: The CAMP method requires both trainers who are experts in the subject matter and peer trainers. In most cases, CDI training will require a pairing of a CDI expert with a peer of the trainees, if possible.

4. Resolution of concerns: After a review of the objectives, trainers should begin every training program by asking the attendees for their concerns and addressing these concerns as best as possible before proceeding with the training.

5. Delivery of information: Trainers deliver the information in a manner that follows the program's objectives. They provide attendees with a handout of the PowerPoint slides or other reference tools, involve trainees in discussions about their own experiences, and encourage questions and concerns throughout the program.

6. A mastering component: To ensure sustainability of the training and obtain the best results, the training program is designed so the trainees have an opportunity to apply the information they are being taught during the training session. There should be at least one opportunity for the trainees to practice during the training session.

7. Coaching: Trainers end the session with encouraging statements regarding the trainees ability to internalize and apply the information they learned during the training session.

8. Evaluation and feedback: The attendees are asked to evaluate the program. The evaluations can be used to improve future sessions and to identify other opportunities for training program topics.

9. Testing: To the extent possible, trainees should be tested on the information they learned during the session.

Post-training Tests

Requiring program attendees to successfully complete a test after a training program has compliance, operational, and even personal benefits. First, from a compliance perspective, having documented evidence of what the organization's staff and the physicians know can be helpful in demonstrating that the management team provided the correct direction, support, and tools to these individuals. Second, because a test is more likely to guarantee the information is retained and used by program attendees, the CDI function will benefit from the operational improvements likely to result. Finally, when trainees know they will need to complete a test after training, they are more likely to focus on the information being taught. At the very least, the trainees will benefit personally from learning a new skill or adding to their information base.

The tests that are easiest to administer are multiple choice. Since the organization is accountable for acting on poor test results, it is best to use an online testing system that allows continuous retakes until the test-taker passes the test. These tests, which are embedded in most e-learning systems, generate subsequent tests with different questions in a different order.

Data from test results can be used in overall program management. Minimally, the results of the test should be shared with the test-taker. However, CDI program managers can also calculate mean scores for trainees overall or by subgroup and use this information in their program reporting. They may want to set targets for mean scores. For example, they may want to set a mean test score at 90 percent and continue to require staff to either retake the random testing instruments (if they have a Web-based testing instrument) or continue to participate in follow-up training until the mean score reaches the minimum target.

Tables 11.2 and 11.3 provide examples of the use of mean test score reporting together with operational and compliance measures for both CDI staff members and physicians. These tables are presented in a report card format and can be used to inform

Table 11.2　CDI specialist report card

Key Indicator	Grade	Achievement	Target	Variance
Doc Spec Fitness Test™ Results	◆◆◆◆◆	92%	90%	102%
Concurrent review productivity	◆◆◆	98%	100%	98%
Documentation review accuracy	◆	87%	98%	89%
Concurrent query rate (records w/queries)	◆◆◆	26%	35%	74%
Total number of queries placed	◆◆◆◆◆	350	325	108%
Concurrent response rate	◆	25%	60%	42%

◆◆◆◆◆ —key indicator results better than expected

◆◆◆ —key indicator results within 10% of expected

◆ —key indicator results

Table 11.3　Medical staff CDI report card

Key Indicator	Grade	Achievement	Target	Variance
Physician CDI Knowledge Assessment	◆	75%	90%	83%
Concurrent Query Rate	◆◆◆	26%	35%	74%
Concurrent Response Rate	◆	25%	60%	42%
Retrospective Query Rate	◆◆◆	7%	12%	58%
Retrospective Response Rate	◆	50%	85%	59%
Documentation Legibility	◆	72%	98%	73%
Documentation Accuracy	◆	50%	90%	56%

◆◆◆◆◆ —key indicator results better than expected

◆◆◆ —key indicator results within 10% of expected

◆ —key indicator results

senior management, the compliance department, and the medical staff of the current strengths of the program as well as areas that need improvement.

Compliance Versus Operations as the Reason for Review and Education

Not every issue identified during CDI program monitoring or during an audit is a compliance issue. In fact, in many cases, problems or concerns are operational in nature. If not corrected, it is possible that some operational issues can become compliance issues. Ultimately, the organization wants the CDI program to be running smoothly from both an operational and a compliance perspective. It also wants the program and its review processes to be as efficient as possible. There is no reason, for example, to conduct CDI department-specific operational reviews differently from reviews used to validate compliance. The organization's compliance department is focused on auditing for compliance purposes. However, it makes the most sense for CDI reviews not conducted by the compliance department to look at any potential issues with the CDI function—compliance, operational, or other. The same is true for educational follow-up. Both operational and compliance issues can be addressed in the same educational session. For example, the same educational program can train the staff or the physicians on how to query in a more compliant manner as well as how to increase the productivity of reviews.

Conclusion

Clinical documentation is the basis of the coding and billing activity in every organization, therefore CDI should be included in the organizational compliance program. CDI program managers can and should organize their internal operations to include policies and procedures, regular monitoring, annual audits, and targeted follow-up education that address both compliance and operational issues. There should be continuous open lines of communication between the CDI program manager and the compliance team. The compliance department should be informed of any possible compliance problems identified within the CDI department. Education that focuses on addressing issues identified during monitoring or auditing should ideally include a follow-up test. Detailed documentation should be created and maintained for all CDI monitoring, audits, and educational program content and attendance.

References

Babbie, E. 1999. *The Basics of Social Research*. Albany, NY: Wadsworth Publishing Company.

Centers for Medicare and Medicaid Services (CMS) and the National Center for Health Statistics (NCHS). 2006a. ICD-9-CM Official Guidelines for Coding and Reporting. www.cdc.gov/nchs/datawh/ftpserv/ftpicd9/ftpicd9.htm.

Centers for Medicare and Medicaid Services (CMS) and the National Center for Health Statistics (NCHS). 2006b. ICD-9-CM Official Guidelines for Coding and Reporting—Supplement. 2006. http://www.cdc.gov/nchs/data/icd9/POAguideSep06.pdf.

Department of Health and Human Services. Office of the Inspector General. 1998. Medicare payments for DRG 475: Respiratory system diagnosis with ventilator support. Washington, D.C. Office of the Inspector General, 1998. (OEI-03-98-00560).

Department of Health and Human Services. Office of the Inspector General. 1999a. Compliance Program Guidance for Hospitals. Washington, D.C. Office of the Inspector General. http://www.oig.hhs.gov/authorities/docs/cpghosp.pdf.

IPRO. 2005a. Coding for Quality: Documentation tips for the Top Seven DRGs Revised 2005, Hospital Payment Monitoring Program. http://providers.ipro.org/index/hpmp.

IPRO. 2005b. Coding for Quality: Documentation tips for the Top Ten Denied DRGs, Hospital Payment Monitoring Program. http://providers.ipro.org/index/hpmp.

Russo, R. and S. Fitzgerald. 2008. Physician Clinical Documentation: Implications for Healthcare Quality and Cost. Academy of Management Annual Meeting, Anaheim, CA.

Wang, M. Q., E. Fitzhugh, and R. C. Westerfield. 1995. Determining sample sizes for simple random surveys. *Health Values* 19(3): 53–56.

Part 3

Growing and Refining the Clinical Documentation Program

Chapter 12
Continual CDI Program Renewal

CDI should be a dynamic function in every organization. The healthcare environment supports continuous renewal of the clinical documentation program. Moreover, CDI is a relatively new function in most organizations. Therefore, changes are likely to occur as a result of the natural development of the program. Examples of activities that create an environment ripe for continuous renewal include:

1. Regulatory changes

2. Training for new medical staff, house staff, and other clinicians

3. Evolution of quality initiatives

4. Expansion of the CDI program into new areas

5. Ongoing refinement of the program with the assistance of the medical staff

Business and personal growth experts have found that continuous renewal, also known as "sharpening the saw," is practiced by organizations and individuals who are the most effective at what they do (Covey 1989; Drucker 1999). This chapter will discuss clinical documentation renewal efforts in terms of how the programs are likely to grow organically. The development of the physician training function and the refinement of program measures are also covered.

Growing the CDI Function

All CDI program implementation is focused, at least initially, on one patient care area: the inpatient setting. The reasons for this are threefold. First, the organization is taking a risk by investing in a new program. By focusing on one area, the risk of failure is minimized. Second, the organization will want to measure return on investment in some meaningful way. Focusing on one area makes this initial measurement more efficient and reliable. Third, targeting one area for CDI allows an organization to develop a successful model that can be replicated or modified to fit the needs of other patient care areas. It also allows the organization to create the building blocks for CDI that can be used to develop other functions such as training and patient education that are synergistic with CDI.

Where an organization takes the CDI function after the initial implementation depends on the organization. However, it is known that allowing a program to stagnate at its original level of implementation will likely result in less support over time from the medical staff (Russo 2008). Lack of medical staff support leads to the inability to reach program targets and the possibility of program dissolution altogether. Table 12.1 is an example of various growth and renewal patterns that a CDI program can take. These are suggestions only as it is essential for every organization to grow the function based on what makes sense for that organization. Basic suggestions about program renewal include:

- Wait until the program has a complete year of stable, successful operations before attempting to expand it.

- Initial expansion should be planned in small steps so as not to detract from the core program. In table 12.1, the initial year of implementation shows the only expansion being the addition of specialty-specific training for physicians as a follow-up to the initial base education all physicians receive.

- In the initial growth years, add services and activities that can be predicted with a high degree of certainty to add value to the organization. This can be determined through pilot studies performed prior to the expansion.

While riskier expansion can often result in big payoffs, this activity should be saved for later years. In table 12.1 some of the less traditional expansions include providing community education to healthcare consumers to train them on the content and use of their health records. The ultimate purpose is to show the direct relationship between clinical documentation and the patient. Natural benefits of this activity might be improved patient satisfaction and even improved alignment with the medical staff, especially if the hospital can involve physicians in training the community about their health records.

Table 12.1   CDI program growth and renewal possibilities

Program Timeline	Operational Activities
Initial Implementation	Inpatient review and querying
	Obtain support and cooperation of the medical staff
	Provide specialty-specific education
Year 2	Add ED and clinic concurrent reviews
	Add quality measures review into annual audit results for inpatients
	All attending physicians trained in documentation principles by end of the year
Year 3	Add ambulatory surgery concurrent reviews
	Begin CDI training for every clinician who documents in a patient record
Year 4	Continue CDI training for every clinician
	Add outpatient testing concurrent reviews
	Create synergy between current clinical education processes (grand rounds, mortality and morbidity review) and clinical documentation principles
Year 5	Offer community training to healthcare consumers to understand their health records; recruit physicians to assist in the process
	Develop a predictive measure between clinical documentation practices and quality measures using first three years of program data
Year 6	Develop a tracking system to measure patients' satisfaction with their health information
	Incorporate patient satisfaction and predictive quality measures into regular program reporting

Developing the CDI Training Sessions for Physicians

Initially, the medical staff may not look forward to the mandatory documentation training sessions provided by the CDI function. However, it should be the goal of every CDI program to develop a rapport with the physicians so that eventually, the medical staff views CDI as a valuable resource they can access for their own benefit.

Position CDI as Value-added

It is important to position the CDI function in a way that the physicians view the services offered by the clinical documentation staff as a value-added service for them (Russo 2003). The following six activities may be used as a way to develop a better understanding of how the CDI function can better serve physicians.

Obtain Feedback from Physicians

The best way to find out how to better serve a customer is to ask. And, physicians are a customer of the clinical documentation function. They also serve as a provider of raw material in the clinical documentation supply chain. But, thinking about them as customers will help to develop the right approach to the ongoing relationship between CDI staff and the medical staff. CDI staff should ask physicians for feedback—verbally, with Web-based surveys, and through service chiefs. They should ask what the physicians do and do not like about the CDI function, what CDI staff can do to facilitate the process for physicians, and how CDI staff can be of better service to physicians in helping to improve their documentation skills overall.

Listen and Observe Physicians

When asking, it is important to listen. CDI staff may find that they can obtain a significant amount of information from physicians by simply listening to the physicians talk—at training functions, during staff meetings, and on the units. Physicians are often quite verbal about what is bothering them. The CDI function is not designed to be a panacea for all physician problems with the hospital. However, if CDI staff learn about a physician issue and can determine how CDI training or support can help, they should act on it. For example, they may have heard a physician mention a problem with the rejection of office bills by a certain payer. The bills are being rejected for medical necessity issues, and neither the physician nor the office staff have been able to manage the situation effectively. While the CDI staff cannot offer their services to analyze and fix the problem for the physician, they can offer education and training that would benefit both the physician's practice and the hospital. There may even be some tools that they have or can develop that they can provide to the physician as a takeaway during the training.

Demonstrate How the Health Record is a Common Ground

The health record is the common ground between the medical staff and the hospital. The medical staff needs the record to treat the patient and communicate with other caregivers. The hospital needs the record to translate its contents into coded data for billing, quality indicators, research, and planning. Telling physicians this will not make them see their responsibility in clinical documentation any differently. However, taking the opportunity to interject the health record topic into physician encounters such as mortality reviews, department meetings, grand rounds, and training programs can help get the message across. Using the health record as a tool to accomplish goals in the hospital will likely encourage the physicians to begin to incorporate the same tools in their day-to-day activities. As the EHR becomes more prevalent, this concept will grow in popularity with physicians. Since many physicians are enamored with technology, pulling together the CDI opportunity with the EHR may increase their curiosities.

Provide Web-based Training and Web-based Resources

Web-based training provides advantages for all staff, not just physicians. Increased productivity, less cost, and greater compliance justify the initial investment (Chung et al. 2004). For organizations that already provide Web-based training, physicians should be asked for feedback about their experience with the tool. If possible, CDI staff should improve the tool to increase physician satisfaction. They can also develop a Web-based resource that provides physicians and their office personnel with information about billing issues that are related to clinical documentation practices. If an organization owns physician practices, chances are it already has these resources for use by the billing staff. Making this type of resource available to physicians could be one more way to see the importance of clinical documentation, especially for billing purposes.

Create Codevelopment Opportunities

Some hospital CDI staff members have begun to partner with their physicians to present the success of their CDI program at local, state, and even national association meetings. This type of codevelopment opportunity can be used to build improved relationships with physicians using the CDI program as a common ground. CDI staff can also work with physicians to design research projects (or even pilots to expand the CDI program) or write papers for publication in academic journals. Physicians, especially those in academic medical centers, have a great interest in having their work published. Any of these activities would bring benefit to both the physician and the organization (Flamholtz and Lacey 1981). The fact that CDI is used as the basis of the activity is likely to make physicians more responsible and accountable for their documentation practices.

Establish a Clinical Documentation Advisory Board (and Pay for Their Time)

This may be a long stretch for many organizations. However, considering the minimal cost to an organization for paying a physician to serve on a board for clinical documentation planning, the benefits far outweigh the expenses. If the organization has an interest in this type of venture, it will need to be explicit about the responsibilities of the physician advisors. The advisory board cannot be like every other committee that physicians may serve on in the hospital, since they are not paid for those activities. The physicians would have additional responsibilities. Perhaps CDI staff can train them to be peer reviewers or trainers for physician CDI training. If the advisory board member service time can be limited to six months or a year, not only would it potentially appeal more to the members, it would also give the organization the opportunity to intensively train several physicians a year in CDI principles. With the right planning, the right physician participants, and the right process the results could prove to be mutually beneficial to the organization and to the physicians.

CDI staff should consult their compliance officer for specific guidance on how to create the advisory board and work with physicians compliantly. There are certain Medicare antitrust laws that prohibit hospitals from giving physicians anything of value that would appear to be an inducement to the physician for admitting patients to the hospital. However, if the hospital is paying the physicians fair market value for actual work performed outside of normal hospital duties, this should not be a problem. The activity should be overseen by the organization's compliance team or general counsel's office.

Specialty-specific Training

After all physicians (or some acceptable target percentage of physicians) have been trained in the baseline CDI education, it is important to begin developing specialty-specific training. A physician CDI advisory board, is the perfect place to begin creating the programs with the assistance of the physicians on the board. In creating the sessions, CDI staff will want to obtain feedback from physicians in each specialty. They should also consider using service-specific patient records from the hospital in all educational programs. Creating ongoing educational programs that use the case study method will make it easier for physicians to learn because they are accustomed to this technique.

Professional Fee Training

Training physicians about how their documentation in patient records impacts their professional fee reimbursement can be a key benefit to the physician. In addition, this training can result in being a prime benefit to the hospital if additional physicians cooperate because they appreciate the hospital providing them with this information (Russo 2001). Figures 12.1 and 12.2 show examples of hospital progress notes that can be used to demonstrate how documentation added to the hospital record to bring the note into compliance for high-quality clinical documentation also impacts the physician's professional fee billing for the hospital visit. During these training sessions, it is best to have a physician professional fee coding and billing expert available to answer specific questions that physicians may pose. Providing this expert resource for the physicians during the training can be viewed as an additional benefit to them, and it will hopefully result in higher levels of support and cooperation from the physicians for the CDI program.

Figure 12.1   Sample hospital progress note (also used for physician professional fee billing)

Progress Note: Admitted through ED for generalized abd pain, dehydration
Old records: Requested, reviewed
      Heart: RRR, carotid pulses
      Lungs: CTA
      ABD: soft, NT, BS normal, no hemorrhoids
RLQ tenderness, guarding
A/P: RLQ abd, pain, dehydration

Additional "query" diagnosis: ETOH abuse or intoxication on admission based on blood alcohol levels upon admission, but not documented.

Figure 12.2   Sample hospital progress note (also used for physician professional fee billing)

Progress Note: No complaints, Hx bleeding ulcer 2 yrs. ago
Labs: WBC-10.5   Hemoglobin-10.5   Hematocrit-30.6
      Heart: RRR
      Lungs: CTA
      ABD: soft, NT, No HSM, BS normal, CVAT, no hemorrhoids
Small umbilical hernia, easily reducible stools for $\oplus$ occult blood
A/P: GI bleed, umbilical hernia

Additional "queried" diagnosis: blood loss anemia based on lab values

Refining Program Measures

A final consideration for continuous program renewal is the refinement of program measures. The core CDI key metrics described in prior chapters will always remain in place. However, other metrics can be added or current ones can be modified to spark renewed interest. To the extent that CDI staff can continue to develop measures that show the value that CDI is bringing to the organization, they will want to implement these measures. Some specific ways to think differently about program metrics include:

1. How can the metrics be used to develop physician report cards?

2. Where has CDI had an integrative impact with other functions in the organization and how can those be reported to show greater value to the organization?

3. How does CDI influence quality measures?

4. How has CDI positively impacted physician satisfaction?

5. How has CDI positively impacted patient satisfaction?

Physician Report Cards

One of the easiest measures to create from CDI data is an individual physician report card. The same measures that are collected and reported on regularly for the program can be used to create a measurement tool for physicians. This activity should only be undertaken if it is supported by the medical staff. Otherwise, creating and distributing physician report cards could harm the hospital-physician relationship. Table 12.2 shows an example of a physician report card that includes measures for testing (knowledge assessment), query rates, response rates, documentation legibility (assessed separately at this hospital), and documentation accuracy (determined through an auditing process). The diamonds, which were added to mimic the HealthGrades' graphics, allow the viewer to determine at a glance the documentation quality for each physician. This report card represents poor quality documentation practice as the majority of the grades are lower than expected.

Figure 12.3 is a graph that contains a different version of physician-report-card reporting. In this example, severity is measured by physician against the average length of stay. As previously discussed, lower severity levels are likely to receive lower quality

Table 12.2   Sample physician CDI report card

Key Indicator	Grade	Achievement	Target	Variance
Physician CDI knowledge assessment	◆	75%	90%	83%
Concurrent query rate	◆◆◆	26%	35%	74%
Concurrent response rate	◆	25%	60%	42%
Retrospective query rate	◆◆◆	7%	12%	58%
Retrospective response rate	◆	50%	85%	59%
Documentation legibility	◆	72%	98%	73%
Documentation accuracy	◆	50%	90%	56%

◆◆◆◆◆ —key indicator results better than expected

◆◆◆ —key indicator results within 10% of expected

◆ —key indicator results less than expected

Figure 12.3 Severity of illness and length of stay measures by individual physicians.

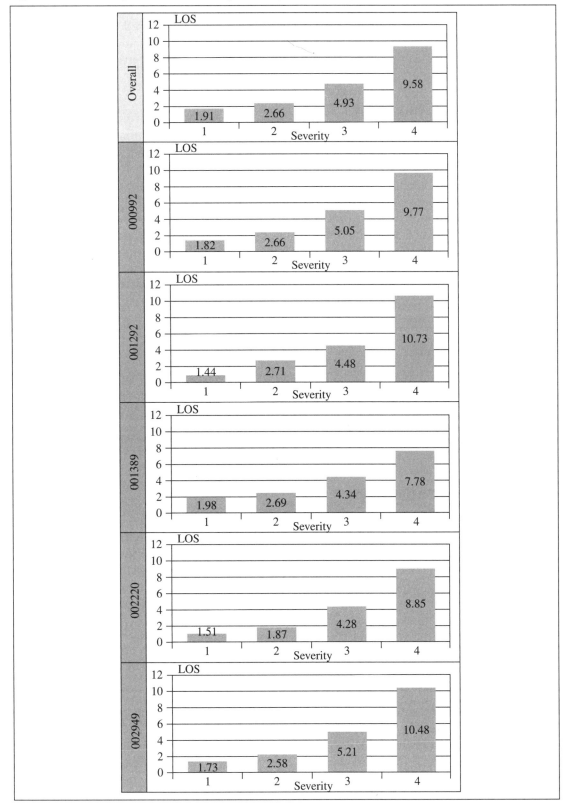

indicators and lower scores on HealthGrades quality reports since severity is a key indicator of quality for these measures. One feature of this report card is that it compares several different physicians. Here, identification numbers are used for each physician. These numbers can be assigned so only the individual physician knows the number, thus preserving anonymity. This type of reporting system may be preferred by some medical staffs.

Integrative Impact of CDI

To the extent that the CDI function interfaces with other functions, it may be determined that the synergies create added benefits to the organization. If this is the case, CDI staff will want to report on that phenomenon. For example, CDI may impact the work of HIM, quality, compliance, patient accounting, and case management functions. When this is suspected, it is important for CDI staff to work together as a team with the managers of these departments to demonstrate that the improved results are coming from synergies that would not exist if either department was acting independently. For example, the CDI specialists may interact with the coding staff on a regular basis. In some organizations, a CDI specialist and a coder are teamed up to discuss cases and follow retrospective queries. The team may find that the retrospective query response rate prior to the teamwork was 50 percent but has now risen to 90 percent. This is a good example of a measure that should be reported.

Quality Impact

As Medicare quality indicators and other quality measures continue to be refined, it is important to clarify the CDI program and the program measures that accompany the quality component. Today, severity of illness is the measure of CDI that most closely impacts severity. As CDI staff identify additional relationships and can demonstrate a positive impact between CDI activities and the quality outcome, they should collect the data and report on the measures.

Physician Satisfaction

As CDI staff position CDI as a value-added service to physicians on the medical staff, it will be important to collect information from them about their attitudes and opinions regarding the program, documentation practices, and the other services they offer. They will want to track these responses internally on an ongoing basis. Once the CDI program has reached the point where it is able to show consistently high levels of physician satisfaction with the services provided by the CDI function, CDI staff should share this information with the appropriate managers in the organization. If possible, the physician satisfaction measure should be included on the organization's dashboard (Carroll and Tansey 2000).

Patient Satisfaction

Today, thinking about the relationship between CDI activities and patient satisfaction is a long stretch. However, as CDI initiatives are able to engage in continuous program renewal, they may have the opportunity to bring documentation to the patients. By providing individuals in the community with training on how to request, use, and read their health records, CDI programs are educating them on their documentation. One way to show the impact that CDI can have on patient satisfaction is to measure patients' responses to training and how it helped them read and interpret their health records. This activity is an important community service, and it can be used to demonstrate to physicians that their documentation practices directly impact not only the care the patient receives, but the patient's overall satisfaction with the healthcare experience.

Conclusion

The healthcare organization should spend a full year implementing a clinical documentation program. At the end of the second year of operations and beyond, it is important to begin refining and renewing the program. Renewal efforts begin with subtle refinements that include physician-specialty training and progress to larger activities that involve expanding CDI into outpatient treatment arenas. The renewal of the program should be viewed as an opportunity to build better relationships with the physicians. Program renewal should include refining program measures, expanding physician training, and positioning the program as a value-added service by the medical staff.

References

Carroll, R. F. and R. R. Tansey. 2000. Intellectual capital in the new internet economy—its meaning, measurement and management for enhancing quality. *Journal of Intellectual Capital*. 1(4):296.

Chung, S., D, Mandl, M. Shannon, and G. R. Fleisher. 2004. Efficacy of an educational Web site for educating physicians about bioterrorism. *Academic Emergency Medicine*. 11(2): 143–146.

Covey, S. 1989. *7 Habits of Highly Effective People*. New York: Free Press.

Drucker, P. 1999. *Management for the 21st Century*. New York: HarperCollins.

Flamholtz, E. G., and J. M. Lacey. 1981. Personnel management: Human capital theory and human resource accounting. *Journal of Industrial Relations*.

Russo, R. 2001. The application of knowledge management principles to compliant coding activities. *Topics in Health Information Management*. 21(3):18–22.

Russo, R. 2008. *A Compelling Case for Clinical Documentation. Use Clinical Documentation to Achieve Strategic Alignment with Your Medical Staff.* (Volume 1). Bethlehem, PA: DJ Iber Publishing.

Chapter 13
CDI Best Practices: Operational and Financial

Without doubt, best practice CDI programs are managed proactively. However, the term, best practices, can be subjective in nature. Because the topic to which it is referring is likely to change over time, so too will some of the best practices change. There are portions of best practices descriptions, however, that remain constant over time. This chapter describes best practices using four criteria:

1. Only those best practices likely to remain constant over time are included.

2. Only those best practices that are supported by research or actual application by more than one healthcare system are included.

3. The practice needs to impact at least two out of three management areas (operations, strategy, and compliance).

4. The practice must provide some measurable value to the organization.

Using these four criteria, the 10 best CDI practices are presented.

Ten Best CDI Operational Practices

Create a Vision

Every CDI program needs a strong vision that both is compelling and is consistent with the organization's overall values, vision, and mission statement. Research has shown that organizations that develop meaningful vision statements are more likely to achieve their goals and are more likely to be profitable (Covey 1989; Collins and Porras 1994; Collins 2001). While a vision statement is strategic in nature, it is also operational when created by CDI managers and staff.

The vision statement is an affirmation of where the CDI program is going. It explains in a brief sentence why the organization is willing to dedicate resources to support the clinical documentation effort. The statement may be as simple as, "The CDI program will ensure our data is of the highest possible quality and, as a result, our healthcare system will have accurate reimbursement, quality measures, and high patient satisfaction with health information." The vision statement is usually paired with a mission statement that explains how the vision will be achieved. In the case of a CDI program, some of the means used to achieve the vision include obtaining physician support and involvement in the program and using the best technology including EHR implementation. As with the organizational vision and mission statement, the CDI vision must be crafted to be specific to the organization. Additional details about developing a viable vision statement for CDI can be found in chapter 5.

Implement Initial Compulsory Physician Education

Compulsory physician education in CDI using a model like the CAMP Method discussed in chapter 7 is probably the single most important activity undertaken to ensure the success of the CDI program. In the author's experience, organizations who believe they can move forward and be successful implementing a clinical documentation program without full support from the medical staff have significantly underestimated the impact physicians have on CDI. In every case, these organizations either abandoned their program or went back to the drawing board and recreated the program from the ground up with physician support the second time around.

Physician documentation is the issue at hand in the CDI program. Not only do physicians need to be trained on the principles of clinical documentation, they also need to take a leadership role in the function. Through training, physicians develop the skills and the confidence to document accurately (Bandura 2000; Cascio et al. 2005). More importantly, they become active participants in the CDI process. This may mean they attend follow-up training sessions, respond more quickly to queries, and are willing to assist with the training of new physicians.

Training staff using an effective adult learning model has been shown to have a positive impact on organizational efficiency and be sustainable over time (Bandura 2000; Cascio et al. 2005; Mulvehill et al. 2005). In addition to increasing operational efficiency, education and training also reduce compliance risk.

Create Policies and Procedures and Require Sign-off

Policies and procedure development may seem mundane, but programs that develop them, even in their most simple and straightforward form, have consistently been more efficient in their processes and more consistent in their data reporting. Not only is it essential to develop the policies and procedures, it is also just as important to require program staff to sign off on them. This shows they understand the documents and agree to abide by them. The creation of policies and procedures requires the authors, who are usually the managers and staff of the CDI program, to really think through their processes. In essence, writing the process down validates the process. Written policies and procedures support operational efficiency and reduce compliance risk.

Maintain Complete Query Documentation

Every organization should apply the same criteria for high-quality clinical documentation to the recording of CDI program activities as it does to the review of clinical documentation. Complete query documentation is maintained for three reasons. First, thorough documentation of program activities makes the staff members more engaged and responsible for their work. In a program that maintains excellent documentation on the query process, staff are involved in maintaining the documentation. They also know that every step they take in the CDI process can be retraced so they are more likely to act consistently and compliantly. Second, the documentation makes physicians more accountable for their responsibilities to the hospital. Physicians know they cannot slip through the cracks in an efficiently run program.

For example, if the CDI program generates regular reports showing outstanding physician queries, the reason for each query, and the query rate by physician or by service, it sends the message that program documentation is impeccable.

The third reason for keeping thorough query documentation is for compliance purposes. Because CDI is the raw material for coding and billing, activity around the function is often scrutinized closely by the government and private payers. In every instance, the program must have the ability to recreate every query it generates. The query paper trail will serve the organization well in the event of an investigation or during regular auditing activities. Assuming that CDI activities are all performed compliantly, the query paper trail will serve to support why the query was asked (there was clinical evidence to support it), how it was asked (not in a leading manner), and how it was responded to by the physician. Without the query paper trail, just as with everything else that the government investigates, lack of documentation (or evidence) will be held against the organization, not in its favor. The organization can protect itself and minimize compliance risk by maintaining complete documentation on all queries (IPRO 2005a; IPRO 2005b; CMS 2006a; CMS 2006b).

Operationalize a Feedback Loop between Denials, Management, and CDI

CDI is an integrative function in every organization. Most organizations embrace this concept in the initial implementation phase. During implementation, members of the organization responsible for functions that should be continuously integrated with CDI generally serve on the CDI committee. This usually includes compliance, finance, HIM, case management, members of the medical staff, data analysts, case mix managers, and EHR staff. However, often after implementation has been successful and formal committees have been dissolved, the managers and representatives retreat to their respective areas. It is the responsibility of the CDI manager to ensure continuous communication with many of these managers. Specifically, the CDI manager should coordinate a feedback loop with each of these functional managers that involves reporting of data from the department to CDI and then from CDI back to the department. The three areas for CDI best practices include operationalization of feedback loops with denials management, compliance, and HIM.

Every organization has a denials management process in place. Ideally, an organization wants to have its bills paid without a denial. In some organizations denial rates are as high as 50 percent (Johnson 2008; Robertson and Dore 2005). Therefore, the need for a function dedicated to managing the process is necessary in most organizations. Denials management may be part of the finance and patient accounting function, or it may be designated as its own function. The CDI manager should seek out the denials manager to discuss how they can help each other. In particular, denials managers should be collecting the reasons for denials, and one of those reasons is, or should be, documentation issues. In these cases, if the CDI manager could be informed of the reasons for denials that were related to documentation, the manager could design a process to provide assistance in preventing those types of denials.

At a minimum, the CDI manager can use the information to educate the staff and even develop follow-up education for the physicians to clarify what types of documentation issues are causing denials and what strategies they need to take to prevent future denials. The CDI manager can then provide the denials manager with information about the training. This illustrates one possible synergistic opportunity between CDI and denials management. In tracking the cause for denials, the managers should expect to see a decrease in denials due to documentation.

Operationalize a Feedback Loop between CDI and Compliance

A second feedback loop that should be put into place is one between CDI and the compliance function. As previously discussed, CDI can present a significant compliance risk to an organization that does not manage the process correctly. One way to keep CDI on track is to keep a regular, open feedback loop between the function and the compliance manager. For example, the CDI program manager should ask for recommendations from the compliance manager that relate to the current OIG work plan or other compliance activities of the organization. In addition, the CDI manager should report results of audits and monitoring to the compliance department regularly. The CDI manager should also see the compliance function as an opportunity to discuss concerns about physicians who may not be cooperating with program staff or who are ignoring queries. If not managed appropriately, these physicians may become disgruntled with the CDI process and file complaints with CMS, the state's attorney general, or even the OIG. The CDI program should be run proactively. Identifying the potential for compliance issues and resolving them before they turn into actual issues is a smart idea for CDI program managers, the organization, and the medical staff. Keeping a close liaison with the compliance department through a formal feedback loop is a good way to manage this risk.

Operationalize a Feedback Loop between HIM and CDI

The last feedback loop that should be in place for a best practice CDI program is between HIM and the CDI program. In some cases, CDI may report into the HIM manager. However, even a formal reporting structure does not guarantee that the right information will be shared among the right individuals. Therefore, it is necessary to ensure that the CDI manager works directly with the HIM manager to obtain data about retrospective physician queries. This includes retrospective queries made both by the coding professionals and by the CDI specialists on the unit that were not responded to before the patient's discharge. This should be a formal reporting loop. In some CDI databases, the coding professionals have the ability to record retrospective queries (IPRO 2005a; IPRO 2005b; CMS 2006a; CMS 2006b). This is ideal, but in the absence of such a computer program, the CDI manager and the HIM or coding manager need to determine a methodology to ensure this information is shared. Another informal feedback loop that can be put into place between the departments is joint educational sessions for the CDI specialists and the coding staff. Joint training cannot take the place of formal reporting, but it provides a strong support for the staff, especially around common frustrations with the query process.

Figure 13.1 demonstrates the feedback loop that should be in place between the CDI function and other integrated functions within the organization. Depending on the organization, other functions may share data with CDI, but denials management, HIM, and compliance are the three that have the greatest synergy and are likely to produce the most significant value to the organization if teamed with CDI.

Design CDI as a Patient-centered Process

The primary reason for the existence of every healthcare system is the patient. Organizations that design their systems around the patient are likely to be more successful than organizations that do not (Penfield et al. 2009). Because CDI is focused on ensuring the best possible documentation in a patient's health record, it is easy to draw some initial analogies between the function and its direct impact on patients, namely quality of patient care. However, there are some additional areas that CDI programs can take advantage of to expand the patient focus of their function. These include increasing the

Figure 13.1   The clinical documentation integrated feedback loop

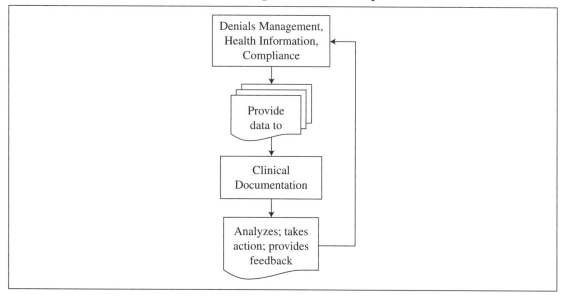

patient's awareness of the health record, assisting the patient to obtain that record, and showing the patient how to read the information in that record. CDI departments have an opportunity to provide information to the community with training or other programs about their health records. This is also an opportunity for the CDI program to work with HIM and members of the medical staff. All three functions together are likely to deliver a better result to patients than an individual one.

Conduct Continuous Targeted Physician Education and Relationship Building

The basic physician education, as noted in the second point is essential to the initial success of a CDI program. However, follow-up education and relationship building are just as essential to the continued success and sustainability of a CDI program. The key to this activity is that the department is not just conducting follow-up education, but doing it in a way that engages the medical staff. The ultimate outcome of physician involvement in the CDI process should be the physicians' perception of CDI as a value-added service to them. Over time, physicians are likely to align themselves naturally with the effort because they see it is in their own best interest and their patients' best interests to practice high-quality clinical documentation.

Use Rigorous Measurement Tools

As mentioned before, an activity not measured cannot be managed. Clinical documentation practices are no exception. As noted in earlier chapters, first the organization develops baseline measures for clinical documentation practices through the assessment. Then, during the course of implementation, the program develops CDI core key metrics targets. Finally, the organization begins to track additional measures as part of its program renewal process. These data must be tracked diligently, analyzed accurately and carefully, and reported to senior management on a regular basis. Current data must be compared against data from an earlier time period to determine whether progress is being made.

In later stages of the life of the CDI program, the organization may want to consider using a Six Sigma process to track and measure program outcomes. Six Sigma is a highly disciplined process that helps to focus on developing and delivering near-perfect products and services. In an organization that practices Six Sigma quality, the goal is to attain a 99.99999 percent accuracy rate. By way of example, the Six Sigma goal in coding is 3.4 defects per one million records coded. Today, it is common for organizations to set a 95 percent proficiency rate for coding. This standard would allow 50,000 defects per million occurrences, far outside the acceptable range for Six Sigma. Although Six Sigma was first practiced in the manufacturing industry, it has been applied to the service industry successfully during the past decade (UVA 2008). Healthcare organizations that have implemented Six Sigma methodologies for improving efficiencies in many different areas have all seen significant financial benefits as a result of the Six Sigma activities (UVA 2008). While a Six Sigma program is likely not part of the initial CDI implementation for every organization, excellent tracking and measuring should be. And, attaining Six Sigma-level quality should be goal for the future.

Five Best Practices for Management of Financial Measures

Because the financial impact of a CDI program is important and because many programs may lose their continued funding without the ability to demonstrate economic value, every organization should have a best practices approach to managing the financial measurement of its CDI program.

Hospital management teams often express concerns related to clinical documentation and case mix index (CMI) management that invoke a compliance, ethics, QIO, or fiscal intermediary-related reason as the cause for nonaction. While apprehension can be understandable given the nature and size of some compliance and fraud and abuse settlements, it is essential for hospitals to manage their financial affairs accurately and proactively. The five best practices are included here.

1. *Track CMI closely and identify real patient mix change.* The CDI program manager should know and understand the organization's patient base and what the true value of the services are that the organization is providing to them. Reporting where possible, for patient admissions, can increase accountability of both the physician and the organization.

2. *Track and report on CC capture rates across the organization and by service.* Concurrent intervention through a clinical documentation program ensures documentation is reflective of care provided. The resulting complete and accurate documentation will result in good information to be translated into coded data by the hospital's coding staff. If the hospital is confident in its data, because monitoring and auditing of the process is in place, then complication and comorbidity (CC) capture rates that exceed the mean or norms should not be a concern.

3. *Know the benchmarks and validate the data regularly.* Benchmarks for CMI, CC capture rate, and DRG pairs are published nationally and by regional quality improvement organizations (QIOs). These benchmarks are meant to be generalized guides to data reporting outcomes. Each hospital's outcomes may be different. Regular internal or external audits should be used to validate documentation and coding. If the hospital's outcomes are higher or lower than the benchmarks and the work has been done to prove the data is valid, then the program should not be concerned with managing to the benchmarks.

4. *Do the right thing for the most accurate data outcome.* A concurrent process will ensure completeness and quality but if, through an audit process, any inaccuracies in documentation or coding are discovered, the CDI program manager should consider the pros and cons of retrospective rebilling and decide along with the right people on the CDI team what approach to take. Proactive management of the hospital's relationship with the QIO and fiscal intermediary (FI) will likely pave the way to adequately address any legitimate retrospective rebilling issues the hospital may encounter.

5. *Create a concurrent documentation process with physician leadership.* Ensuring accurate clinical documentation is a specific practice just as the practice of medicine is. Physicians are not currently taught how to document accurately in medical school or residency. They are not taught the seven criteria for high-quality clinical documentation. They are also not taught the "language of medicine" as it relates to coded data, reimbursement, or quality measures. It is the hospital's responsibility to teach and monitor clinical documentation practices.

Table 13.1 summarizes the best practices for management of clinical documentation financial measures.

Best Practices in Relationship Building for Financial Managers Concerning CDI

The five best practices are essential to managing a hospital's clinical documentation and case mix index. The relationships the hospital financial management team builds inside and outside of the organization will have just as much impact on the success of the hospital's fiscal management that is driven by clinical documentation practices. The hospital's financial management team should ensure proactive management of relationships with the following:

1. The QIO

2. Fiscal intermediary

3. Primary insurers

The hospital should manage relationships with all payers proactively, not just when the payer, FI or QIO show up for an audit or question a bill. Building relationships and sharing necessary information will also strengthen the credibility of the hospital in the eyes of these organizations. In each case, the hospital management team must delegate responsibility and ultimate accountability for relationship management for each entity to a specific individual in the hospital.

Table 13.1 Best practices for managing clinical documentation

Best Practices Approach to Management
Track CMI closely and identify real patient mix change
Track and report on CC rates overall and by service
Know the benchmarks and validate the data regularly
Do the right thing for the most accurate data outcome
Create a concurrent process with physician leadership

Conclusion

The 10 best CDI operational practices and 5 best practices for the management of financial measures were outlined for consideration by healthcare organizations.

Best practices for CDI presented in this chapter were identified through the use of certain criteria. In order for a practice to be considered a best practice for CDI, it needed to be timeless, bring value, and be performed by at least a few organizations that operate successful and sustainable CDI programs. And, the practice had to benefit the system in at least two of the following three areas: operations, strategy, and compliance.

References

Bandura, A. 2000. *Handbook of Principles of Organizational Behavior.* E. A. Locke, Ed. Oxford, England: Blackwell.

Cascio, B. M., J. H. Wilkens, M. C. Ain, C. Toulson, and F. J. Frassica. 2005. Documentation of acute compartment syndrome at an academic healthcare center. *Journal of Bone and Joint Surgery.* 87 (2):346.

Centers for Medicare and Medicaid Services (CMS) and the National Center for Health Statistics (NCHS). 2006a. ICD-9-CM Official Guidelines for Coding and Reporting. www.cdc.gov/nchs/datawh/ftpserv/ftpicd9/ftpicd9.htm.

Centers for Medicare and Medicaid Services (CMS) and the National Center for Health Statistics (NCHS). 2006b. ICD-9-CM Official Guidelines for Coding and Reporting—Supplement. 2006. http://www.cdc.gov/nchs/data/icd9/POAguideSep06.pdf.

Collins, J. 2001. *Good to Great: Why Some Companies Make the Leap and Others Don't.* New York: HarperCollins Publishers.

Collins, J., and G. Porras. 1994. Built to Last: Successful Habits of Visionary Companies. New York: HarperCollins Publishers.

Covey, S. 1989. *7 Habits of Highly Effective People.* New York: Free Press.

IPRO. 2005a. Coding for Quality: Documentation tips for the Top Seven DRGs Revised 2005, Hospital Payment Monitoring Program. http://providers.ipro.org/index/hpmp.

IPRO. 2005b. Coding for Quality: Documentation tips for the Top Ten Denied DRGs, Hospital Payment Monitoring Program. http://providers.ipro.org/index/hpmp.

Johnson, R. M. 2008. Denial management in a clinical laboratory setting. *Clinical Leadership and Management Review.* 22(3).

Mulvehill, S., G. Schneider, C.M. Cullen, S. Roaten, S.,B. Foster, B., and A. Porter. 2005. Template-guided versus undirected written medical documentation: A prospective, randomized trial in a family medicine residency clinic. *Journal of the American Board of Family Practice.* 18:464–469.

Penfield, S., K. M. Anderson, M. Edmund, and M. Belanger. 2009. Toward Health Information Liquidity: Realization of Better, More Efficient Care from the Free Flow of Information. http://www.boozallen.com/publications/article/40808744?lpid=66005

Robertson, B., and A. Dore. 2005. Six steps to an effective denials management program. *Journal of the Healthcare Financial Management Association.* 59(9):82–86,88.

UVA 2008. University of Virginia (UVA) Medical Center Reduces Coding Errors with Six Sigma. Report On Medicare Compliance. http://healthcare.isixsigma.com/library/ content/c030501a.asp.

Chapter 14
Synergies with the Electronic Health Record

Introduction

The majority of U.S. hospitals are in the early stages of the electronic health record (EHR) transformation. The Healthcare Information Management and Systems Society (HIMSS) divides EHR transformation into eight stages with stage 0 being the lowest level of transformation and stage 7 being the highest level. These stages correspond to the activities that healthcare organizations are most likely to undertake in logical sequence when implementing an EHR. HIMSS estimates that as of the third-quarter of 2008, about 17 percent of U.S. hospitals were at stage 0 (HIMSS 2007). Stage 0 means that some clinical automation may be present, but all three of the major ancillary department systems for laboratory, pharmacy, and radiology are not implemented. Roughly 13 percent of hospitals are still in stage 1, 33 percent are in stage 2, 33 percent are in stage 3, 2 percent are in stage 4, 1 percent are in stages 5 and 6 respectively. And, less than 1 percent of hospitals in the HIMSS analytics database were at stage 7 at the time the study was conducted. Stage 7 means the hospital has a paperless shared electronic health record (SEHR) environment with a mixture of discreet data, document images, and medical images. The criteria for each stage builds upon the prior stages. In order to be in stage 4, the hospital had to have achieved all requirements for stages 0 through 3 first, or concurrently with stage 4 transformation activities. The data show the strongest correlations between higher quality indicators and hospitals that have reached at least stage 4 on their EHR scores (HIMSS 2005). A stage 4 EHR means the hospitals have the following in place:

- All three of the major ancillary clinical systems (pharmacy, laboratory, radiology) are installed and feed data to a central data repository (CDR) that provides physician access for retrieving and reviewing results.

- The CDR contains a controlled medical vocabulary and the clinical decision support and rules engine for rudimentary conflict checking.

- Clinical documentation (vital signs, flow sheets) is required. Nursing notes, care plan charting, and the electronic medication administration record (eMAR) system are scored with extra points and are implemented and integrated with the CDR for at least one service or one unit in the hospital.

- Computerized practitioner/physician order entry (CPOE) for use by any clinician is added to the nursing and CDR environment along with the second level of clinical decision support capabilities related to evidence-based medicine protocols. If one patient service area has implemented CPOE and has completed the previous stages, then this stage has been achieved (HIMSS 2005).

An analysis of the stages of EHR implementation reveals several opportunities for synergies between EHR implementation and CDI. This chapter will use the stages of EHR implementation to identify opportunities for synergy with CDI that are likely to bring added value to the organization. All hospitals with at least 100 beds have median scores of 2.0, which means they have implemented the EHR through stage 2. In addition, stage 2 is considered the foundation stage for implementing more sophisticated EHRs. Because the focus is on the opportunities for CDI synergies during EHR implementation, this analysis will begin with stage 3 and continue through stage 7 (HIMSS 2005).

The biggest challenge with clinical documentation and the EHR is achieving a balance between the technology demands and the need for physician input to ensure that, with the right input, the system produces useful, high-quality information (Fichman and Moses 1999; Goldberg 2000). Involving the medical staff in the process from the beginning is the only way to accomplish this operational goal. Furthermore, understanding what matters to the physicians for patient care and for their own practices and joining this with what the hospital needs for care, reimbursement, research, and planning is the ultimate strategic goal. Everyone including the patient, the physician, and the healthcare organization will benefit from these collaborations.

CDI Opportunities at Stage 3 EHR Implementation

Stage 3 transformation means that clinical documentation (vital signs, flow sheets) is required. Nursing notes, care plan charting, and the electronic medication administration record (eMAR) system are scored with extra points and are implemented and integrated with the CDR for at least one service or one unit in the hospital. The first level of clinical decision support is implemented to conduct error checking with order entry (drug/drug, drug/food, drug/lab conflict checking normally found in the pharmacy). Some level of medical image access from picture archive and communication systems (PACS) is available for access by physicians via the organization's intranet or other secure networks outside of the radiology department confines (HIMSS 2007).

It is essential to involve CDI in the initial stages of CPOE. One of the most common reasons for documentation that fails to meet the criteria for high quality is lack of completeness or precision when an order is placed without a diagnosis or other reason for the order. This applies to orders for diagnostic testing as well as medication. In every instance, the physician should be required to enter a reason for the order. Depending on what is known at the time of the order, the reason may be a symptom, a condition listed as rule out, or an established diagnosis (Pepper 1995).

It is important that documentation practices are considered prior to CPOE being implemented. Consideration of the need for documentation to meet the quality criteria may mean, for example, that the EHR includes a drop-down menu that provides physicians with choices, including the ability to enter free text. Or, an organization may decide that only free text is permissible. The healthcare system's compliance function as well as CDI should be involved in the implementation of the EHR. The involvement of both functions will ensure not only that the criteria for high-quality clinical documentation are met, but also that the methodology used is a compliant one. There are so many opportunities to pull forward, copy, or check off information in the EHR that specific checks as well as training protocols need to be built into the use of every EHR system.

CDI Opportunities at Stage 4 EHR Implementation

Stage 4 means that there is a CPOE system for use by any clinician along with the second level of clinical decision support capabilities related to evidence-based medicine protocols. If one patient service area has implemented CPOE and completed the previous stages, then this stage has been achieved (HIMSS 2007).

Stage 4 involves both full CPOE implementation and decision support related to evidence-based medicine protocols. The organization should continue to work with CDI and CPOE implementation in the same manner as described in stage 3 transformation. The use of computerized evidence-based medicine protocols presents additional opportunities for value-added synergies between EHR implementation and CDI. There are a few ways to accomplish this.

First, educational programs can be developed that explain the relationship between evidence-based medicine and clinical documentation. Examples of how the practice of high-quality clinical documentation can help achieve evidence-based medicine, or at least the legitimate documentation of it, can be emphasized throughout the training. Evidence-based medicine is a concept that appeals to most physicians because they are trained as scientists. Showing a relationship between evidence-based medicine and clinical documentation practices can strengthen support from the physicians for the CDI program (Brown et al. 2005; Timmermans and Berg 2003). More importantly, if physicians believe their clinical documentation practices can have an effect on the practice of medicine through evidence-based medicine protocols, they will be more likely to incorporate high-quality criteria into their clinical documentation practices.

Second, the CDI function should work closely with the organization's protocol management software vendor, if they have one. There are several software programs available to ensure the provider abides by established evidence-based medicine practices. Evidence-based medicine software provides medical practitioners with access to the latest treatment guidelines and protocols at the point-of-service. By centralizing this information and automating its delivery, the software enables healthcare institutions to comply with the demanding requirements of evidence-based medicine and achieve high standards of consistency and quality in dispensing patient treatment (Donaldson and Lohr 1994). In cases where it is possible to create organization-specific queries, the CDI function should be involved. Here, the CDI staff can identify, for example, documentation issues that may be common queries for certain diagnoses and incorporate these into the program as reminders for the physicians. This process, if it is designed properly and if physicians receive thorough training on it, can result in improved quality of documentation as well as a compliant process.

Third, the CDI program manager should ensure that criteria for high-quality clinical documentation are included in any clinical guidelines used by the organization, even if a software program is not currently being used by the organization. Some of the purposes of evidence-based medicine include the ability to inform medical staff of current treatment guidelines and procedures as well as to ensure protocol adherence and regulatory compliance. The treatment guidelines are a convenient place to include the seven criteria for high-quality clinical documentation as a constant reminder for physicians. It is a good idea to reinforce high-quality clinical documentation criteria with the physicians beginning with their exposure to the criteria in the CDI physician training, follow up training, and reporting of key metrics, and extending into as many day-to-day encounters that the physicians have with the patient record. The CDI program manager should identify every possible opportunity to build the criteria for high-quality clinical documentation into existing and new systems, such as the EHR.

Finally, by the time stage 4 transformation has been achieved, the CDI function should have worked with the EHR team to design a methodology to alert the attending physician whenever an abnormal test result is produced. This process can be cumbersome if not managed appropriately. In teaching hospitals, the responsibility for the review and documentation of abnormal test results is delegated to residents. In other organizations, the CDI specialists may be charged with determining whether the clinical significance of an abnormal test result was documented by the physicians and then querying accordingly. Ultimately, by the time stage 6 is achieved, the EHR should have worked out a methodology for electronically capturing documentation for the clinical significance of abnormal test results (Skuteris 1999). This may be through a template designed specifically for this purpose. Figure 14.1 demonstrates the importance of documenting the clinical significance of abnormal test results as well as the EHR opportunity to alert physicians during stage 4 transformation.

CDI Opportunities at Stage 5 EHR Implementation

Stage 5 transformation means the closed-loop, medication-administration environment is fully implemented in at least one patient care service area. The data flows of the CPOE, pharmacy, and the eMAR applications are tightly coupled and integrated with bar coding technology (or radio-frequency identification [RFID] technology) for the nurse, patient, and medication to support the five rights of medication administration, thereby maximizing point-of-service patient safety processes (HIMSS 2007).

Figure 14.1   Relationship between abnormal test results and the EHR

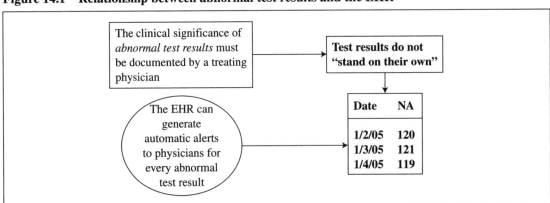

The five rights of medication administration are:

1. Right patient

2. Right route

3. Right dose

4. Right time

5. Right medication (Pepper 1995)

It is interesting to note that in one state department of health's description of the five rights of medication administration, the sentence following the statement of rights was the following: "Ultimately, the appropriate *documentation* should occur as well (DORA 2008)." This is just one example of how medication administration is closely tied to high-quality documentation. Some of the documentation is the physician's, but much of the documentation responsibility belongs to the nursing staff. As noted earlier in the book, every clinician who documents in the patient record should be trained in the principles of high-quality clinical documentation. Synergies with the EHR create the perfect opportunity to get CDI in front of every clinician in the organization.

The closed-loop medication administration includes CPOE plus bar coding, automated dispensing cabinets and robots, and smart infusion pumps. In each step of this process, there are several documentation requirements. For example, step 1 in the CPOE process is to obtain the patient's medication-related history. Steps in the closed loop medication administration related to CDI include the education of both staff and patient regarding the medication, and documentation of the administration and the patient's response to medication.

CDI Opportunities at Stage 6 EHR Implementation

Stage 6 transformation means full physician documentation and charting (using structured templates) is implemented for at least one patient care service area. Level three of clinical decision support provides guidance for all clinician activities related to protocols and outcomes in the form of variance and compliance alerts. A full complement of radiology PACS systems provides medical images to physicians through the Intranet and displaces all film-based images (HIMSS 2007).

Stage 6 transformation of the EHR provides a huge opportunity to solidify CDI concepts in ways and places that the program may not have yet reached. First, the CDI function should be closely involved in template development as well as education on usage. Template design should include requirements for documentation that are clear, consistent, complete, reliable, and where possible, precise. There may be some boiler-plate criteria that are common in all template development. However, each organization should use data from its CDI program reporting to determine specific edits and checks that may need to be built into electronic templates.

Second, stage 6 transformation can incorporate documentation for quality indicators in templates for the physician. The organization can also work with the EHR vendor to develop alerts for missing documentation for quality indicators. This is also a time to revisit the alerts for abnormal test results that were discussed during stage 4 transformation. If any alerts were omitted or if any are not working correctly, they should be repaired by the time the organization achieves stage 6.

Third, stage 6 transformation may be a perfect time for intensive focus on the documentation practices of diagnostic medicine physicians, like radiologists, nuclear medicine physicians, pathologists, and even cardiologists and neurologists involved in interpreting tests like EKGs and EEGs. The impact of improved documentation practices in these areas and the value to the organization extends into almost every patient care setting. At a minimum, this includes not only the inpatient environment, but also the emergency department, ambulatory surgery, outpatient diagnostic testing, and clinics. Simply training the physician diagnosticians on the definition of high-quality clinical documentation may have an impact on content of radiology, MRI, nuclear medicine, and other diagnostic reports.

When educating diagnostic physicians on CDI practices, it is necessary for the CDI staff to stay in the realm of clinical documentation practices only. It is not the role of CDI to judge or make recommendations for diagnosing. This remains the physician diagnostician's responsibility. However, to the extent that these physicians can be trained using examples of their diagnostic reports in patient records where there was either a lack of consistency with the attending physician's documentation or a lack of diagnostic precision, it may help the diagnostician understand the significance of the documentation on the report and the extent to which that documentation is relied upon by others (Bandura 2000; Lenz and Shortridge-Baggett 2002, 143). In all training, the CDI staff's role is to give physicians the criteria with examples and allow them to apply those criteria to their thought process as they are viewing results and dictating reports. It is particularly important for the CDI staff to be cautious with diagnosticians because most do not see the patient and the test results and documentation is the sum total of the encounter. It is even more important that the CDI training for diagnosticians remains focused on the criteria for high-quality clinical documentation because the diagnostician's documentation cannot be relied upon for coding. However, it is important to inform diagnosticians that their documentation can and should be used as essential evidence for queries in relation to the attending physician's documentation.

CDI Opportunities at Stage 7 EHR Implementation

Stage 7 transformation means the hospital has a paperless shared electronic health record (SEHR) environment with a mixture of discreet data, document images, and medical images. Clinical information can be readily shared via electronic transactions or exchange of electronic records with all entities within a regional health information network (other hospitals, ambulatory clinics, subacute environments, employers, payers, and patients) to access healthcare data. This stage allows the healthcare organization (HCO) to support the true integrated care electronic health record (ICEHR) as envisioned in the ideal model (HIMSS 2007).

Stage 7 transformation supports the extension of CDI into areas beyond inpatient, if that has not already occurred. Many of the documentation rules created for templates and CPOE should remain fixed to the clinical documentation modules for outpatient and long-term care service areas. As a result, the means for achieving high-quality clinical documentation in these settings is already in place with the EHR. However, it is still necessary to provide basic education and training to physicians and clinicians in patient care settings where the EHR is migrating. At a minimum, these practitioners should receive training on the principles of clinical documentation and the criteria for high-quality clinical documentation. This training, coupled with documentation rules already in the EHR system should produce good documentation outcomes for the organization.

A second benefit of stage 7 transformation is that it makes health information available to the patient. Prior chapters discussed improved patient satisfaction as an outcome measure for clinical documentation, particularly once more patients begin reviewing the content of their health records. The percentage of patients who review the content of their records is likely to increase after a stage 7 EHR transformation is complete because patients will have access to their EHR without needing to request the information (Tang and Newcomb 1998, 563). Patient satisfaction with their health information brings CDI to a whole new level. It opens the door for the CDI staff to train the community about how to use and understand the EHR. It also makes healthcare providers more accountable to patients for the content of the EHR. The EHR places the hospital, the medical staff, and the patients all behind the need for high-quality clinical documentation, and its achievement appears likely in all patient care settings, with the EHR as the catalyst, as long as healthcare organizations seize the opportunity to incorporate clinical documentation rules into the EHR as described in this chapter.

EHR, Documentation, and Compliance

The focus in this chapter has been on the strategic opportunities to synergize CDI opportunities with each stage of an organization's EHR implementation. Any change brings risks if it is not managed appropriately. In the EHR environment, it is essential to disconnect documentation from coding and charge events which can otherwise present compliance risks to the organization (Trites 2008). In particular, because documentation in an EHR can be cut and pasted and carried forward, along with other compliance concerns, it is essential to ensure that a member of the compliance team is involved in the entire EHR implementation process, as well as the part of the process involving clinical documentation practices.

Conclusion

Significant opportunities exist for synergies between the EHR and improving clinical documentation practices. Different opportunities exist at each of the eight stages of implementation. Most hospitals and healthcare systems have reached level 2 EHR transformation. Therefore, the activities with the most impact and value for the organization can be found in stages 3 through 7 EHR transformation. Each stage provides the possibility for education to all clinicians. However, an organization's CDI experts can also identify documentation improvement opportunities in template development, CPOE design, closed loop medication administration, and extension of the EHR to ancillary services such as radiology, as well as to the patients themselves.

References

Bandura, A. 2000. *Handbook of Principles of Organizational Behavior.* E. A. Locke, ed. Oxford, England: Blackwell.

Brown, M. M., C. G. Brown, and S. Sharma. 2005. *Evidence-Based to Value-Based Medicine.* Chicago: American Medical Association Press.

Carroll-Barefield, A., and L. H. Prince. 2000. Management implications of the health insurance portability and accountability act. *The Health Care Manager* 19(1):44–49.

Donaldson, M., and Lohr, K., eds. 1994. *Health Data in the Information Age.*

Washington, DC: National Academy Press.

DORA. The five rights of medication administration. Colorado Department of Regulatory Agencies. http://www.dora.state.co.us/nursing/news/TheFiveRights.pdf.

Fichman, R. G., and S. C. Moses. 1999. An incremental process for software implementation. *Sloan Management Review.* 40(2):39–52.

Goldberg, I. V. 2000. Electronic medical records and patient privacy. *The Health Care Manager.* 18(3):63–69.

HIMSS. 2005. EMR Sophistication Correlates to Hospital Quality Data: Comparing EMR Adoption to Care Outcomes at UHC Hospitals, Including Davies Award Winners, Using HIMSS Analytics' EMR Adoption Model Scores. HIMSS Analytics White Paper. http:www.himssanalytics.org.

HIMSS. 2007. HIMSS Analytics Database (derived from the Dorenfest IHDS+ Database). HIMSS Analytics Essentials of the US Hospital IT Market 2007.

Lenz, E. R., and L. M. Shortridge-Baggett. 2002. *Self-Efficacy in Nursing: Research and Measurement Perspectives.* New York: Springer Publishing.

Pepper, G. A. 1995. Understanding and preventing drug misadventures: Errors in drug administration by nurses. *American Journal of Health-System Pharmacy* 52(4):369–373.

Skuteris, L. R. 1999. What strategies can help you sensibly manage patient information? *Nursing Management.* 30(1):8.

Starr, P. 1997. Smart technology, stunted policy: Developing health information networks. *Health Affairs.* 16(3):91–105.

Tang, P. C. and C. Newcomb. 1998. Informing patients: A guide for providing patient health information. *Journal of the American Medical Informatics Association.* 6:563–570.

Timmermans, S., and M. Berg. 2003. *The Gold Standard: The Challenge of Evidence-Based Medicine and Standardization in Health Care.* Philadelphia: Temple University Press.

Trites, P. 2008. *How to Evaluate Electronic Health Record Systems.* Chicago: American Health Information Management Association.

Chapter 15
Growing the Clinical Documentation Improvement Program in All Patient-care Areas

Applying the Criteria for High-quality Clinical Documentation to All Settings

Both the CAMP Method and the seven criteria for high-quality clinical documentation addressed in chapters 1 through 3 apply to all documentation by all clinicians in every patient setting. The CAMP Method and the criteria standardize the practice of clinical documentation. However, there is still a need to design training programs that contain examples specific to each outpatient setting and to allow the trainees to master the practice of documentation in each setting. As seen in chapter 14 on EHR implementation, there is an opportunity to use EHR synergies to expand CDI into all patient settings. The EHR can contain templates and alerts for documentation in every care area. However, there is still a need to create a review process that both will be efficient and will achieve the goals of CDI in the context of each patient setting.

Most organizations are in the beginning phases of expanding CDI to settings outside of acute care. The author has designed outpatient CDI programs for the emergency department (ED), outpatient surgery, outpatient testing, and the physician's office. While there were some common components to them, no two programs were exactly the same. This chapter will discuss examples of CDI training and reviews that have been successfully implemented in healthcare systems. Because outpatient CDI is still in its infancy, the programs will evolve over time. For this reason, only examples and practices have been included that are more likely to stand the test of time because of either their efficiency or added value to the organization. In most sections, CDI training and review principles have been included that are common concerns for every organization. As readers progress through the examples and recommendations, they should keep the unique aspects and needs of their own organizations in mind. In particular, note which activities might need to be implemented differently in the organization because of those unique qualities.

Because the most significant amount of clinical documentation per patient occurs in the inpatient setting, many organizations focus their CDI program on inpatient records. However, clinical documentation and its impact permeate every patient-care setting. Most healthcare in the United States occurs in the outpatient setting (NAMCS 2006). In 2003, the most recently-available comprehensive data on healthcare visits, there were 906 million physician office visits, 94.6 million visits to hospital outpatient departments, and 113.9 million ED visits (NAMCS 2006). That same year, there were 34.9 million inpatient hospital discharges (excluding normal newborns). In 2003, therefore, there were approximately 1.1 billion outpatient visits in the United States compared to approximately 35 million inpatient visits to acute care hospitals (NHDDS 2008). Because physician visits are responsible for 80 percent of all outpatient visits, especially if the healthcare system employs or owns physician groups, the importance of high-quality clinical documentation is clear.

Although most organizations begin a CDI initiative in the inpatient arena because of the complexity and amount of documentation, depending on how the organization is structured and its strategic approach to the program, it may begin its CDI program across several different patient-care settings. For example, if structured by product line, the organization may decide to first focus on the cardiology product line. This strategy would involve quality initiatives for documentation in the inpatient cardiac units, the cardiac catheterization laboratory, cardiac rehabilitation programs, and the cardiology groups employed by the organization. The initial investment in this process is much higher than rolling out a program by setting. However, once the program has been implemented across one product line, the ease of implementation across others increases. Although this strategy is not the most common, the ability to build strong physician alliances is greater than when implementing a program by patient setting.

Tailoring CDI Training for the Outpatient Setting

The primary difference between CDI training in the acute care setting and other settings is the examples that are used to teach physicians the mastery part of the documentation process. Most organizations have created CDI training tailored to the inpatient setting using inpatient examples. It is possible, but not optimal, for physicians to learn from inpatient examples and apply the concepts in every setting. Rather, creating examples from each outpatient setting is best. When constructing examples for use in outpatient CDI training programs, issues such as those discussed in the following sections must be considered.

Identify the Most Significant Documentation Challenges for Each Setting

There are some common documentation problems specific to each patient-care setting. However, each organization should assess documentation by setting and identifying documentation issues specific to its facility and practitioners. For example, one common documentation problem in the ED is the use of differential diagnoses or documentation of possible causes or diagnoses to be ruled out in addition to the symptoms. Documentation of diagnoses, if possible, is especially important for patients who are admitted through the ED into the inpatient setting. For short-stay patients admitted through the ED, emergency room physician documentation can be the key to patient care (NACHRI 2007).

Not all ED patients are admitted to the inpatient setting. Therefore, the ED record needs to stand on its own from a documentation perspective. Some ED documentation challenges may include the documentation of reasons for tests and medication orders. If a patient is admitted to the ED and is already on a medication, the diagnosis should be documented as well. If that patient is evaluated for the condition, although it may not be the main reason for admission, this should be documented so it can be captured by the coding staff.

In addition, the OIG has identified medical necessity as a significant issue in most nonacute patient-care areas. Medical necessity audits conducted by the OIG have linked documentation or lack of documentation as the cause for many denials of payment. According to CMS, a claim that requests payment for medically-unnecessary services intentionally seeks reimbursement for a service that is not warranted by the patient's current and documented medical condition (CMS 2006; HHS 1998). This official statement about medical necessity directly links the physician's documentation as the primary indicator of whether a patient's service is medically necessary. Further, the OIG goes on to state that the failure of hospital staff to document items and services rendered is a major area of potential fraud and abuse in federal healthcare programs. The HHS statement goes on to say, "Upon request, a hospital should be able to provide documentation, such as patients' health records and physicians' orders, to support the medical necessity of a service that the hospital has provided" (HHS 1999). These statements continue to justify the need to train all staff in all patient-care settings on high-quality clinical documentation practices.

Utilize Unique Documentation Examples for Each Setting

It is most important in the training to use actual examples from each setting. The CDI trainers should obtain cases that emphasize the uniqueness and the particular documentation challenges of the setting so the physicians and clinicians can recognize the records as their own. All identifiers, especially for the providers, should be deleted from the training materials to avoid embarrassment. The training should be perceived as positive, not a punishment. The trainers should share a few examples of documentation problems and apply the criteria for high-quality clinical documentation to the cases during the lecture. Then, the trainees should be given sample cases and be asked to identify any documentation problems and discuss how they would document the cases differently. This process of applying the concepts learned is important to the sustainability of the training.

Include Template Documentation in Examples

Templates are used in most outpatient settings. They have advantages and disadvantages. Examples should identify cases that make good use of the template and those where documentation can be less than optimal. The OIG in particular looks for templates where documentation for multiple patients is exactly the same. Usually this involves the use of check boxes where the same boxes are checked off for several consecutive patients. The likelihood of identical patient documentation is low. Therefore, when templates contain the same information, this points to a problem with either physician documentation practices or the template design (Khoury et al. 1998). Physician documentation practices can be addressed during the educational settings.

Find 10 Problematic Documentation Examples for Each Setting

The CAMP Method study used 10 case studies when training physicians in the basic principles of high-quality clinical documentation. Because of the study outcome, this number can be viewed as a best practice for physician documentation training. A CDI program may not be able to work the use of 10 case studies into every physician training session, but over the first year, the physicians and clinicians in nonacute settings should be exposed to 10 example cases in subsequent training sessions. As an added tool, Web-based programs may be designed for outpatient CDI training. Documentation examples can be scanned into the training modules so that physicians receive benefit of applying or mastering the CDI process.

Prepare the CDI staff or train locally

Most organizations that have extended clinical documentation functions into the out-patient areas rely upon their CDI team, who likely began the program in the inpatient setting, to perform the work in the outpatient arena. This is especially true for clinical documentation training for physicians and clinicians. CDI program staff who are already experts in training physicians on the criteria for high-quality clinical documentation are generally the best individuals to conduct this training in all settings. Further, the query and data collection process in each outpatient area can be performed by CDI program staff. Or, if it is more geographically convenient, local staff in each outpatient area can be trained to review documentation when and where possible. In each case, additional training in CDI documentation review and data collection (similar to that addressed in earlier chapters) is required.

Designing the CDI Review for the Outpatient Setting

The methodology for CDI concurrent review in the acute care setting is consistent and standardized throughout the healthcare industry. However, the same cannot be said for CDI reviews in the outpatient setting. Clinical documentation teams have developed the process for concurrent inpatient reviews using the structure and staffing in the hospital setting as the venue for the work. Reviewers must do the same in outpatient settings. The following are suggestions for creating an effective review process in alternative patient-care settings. In each setting, the issues have been addressed of who should perform the review, when and where the review should be performed, how it should be performed, and how feedback should be provided to physicians. The same core key metrics should be collected for outpatient CDI as those discussed in earlier chapters. As with all CDI interventions, the key pieces of information are how often documentation is identified that does not meet the criteria for high-quality clinical documentation, who the physician authors of that documentation are, and whether they responded to inquiries to correct their documentation. Other measures may also be collected, depending on the organization. However, these core key metrics should be the minimum measurements for every CDI program regardless of the setting.

Emergency Department

Because many patients are admitted from the ED to the inpatient setting, the ED often is the second patient location where the CDI program is implemented. The CDI staff members have had regular opportunities to review ED documentation during their con-current review of inpatient records (for those patients who were admitted through the ED). Therefore, there usually is a good sense for the specific documentation issues that need to be addressed. Even in this case, the organization should perform a CDI assess-ment for ED records to ensure all relevant issues are identified.

In the ED, physician intervention for CDI should occur prior to discharge. However, every ED will vary in terms of how and if this intervention can occur. The documenta-tion process needs to work around the emergent needs of the patient. The ED is a good location for the use of templates, documentation tools, and EHR documentation alerts. In many hospitals, a case manager controls patient flow in the ED. Therefore, in some instances, outpatient-CDI functions in the ED can be woven into the case manager's existing duties. Specific tools can be designed for use with physicians in the ED to guide their documentation for both facility-based and physician professional fee coding and billing.

Figure 15.1 shows a summary report from a preliminary ED CDI assessment. The report shows the activities that occurred during the assessment as well as recommendations for implementing a CDI program for the ED. The summary provides some ideas as to the specific activities that might be included in an initial CDI assessment in the ED setting.

Ambulatory Surgery and Specialized Procedures

Outpatient surgery and procedures performed in specialized units such as interventional radiology and the cardiac catheterization laboratory each need to be addressed based upon the structure of each unit. Similar to the initial ED assessment previously mentioned, it is necessary to understand the flow of patients and information to determine where the CDI function might be placed. Since time is limited in the outpatient setting,

Figure 15.1   Emergency medicine CDI assessment summary

Emergency Medicine CDI Assessment Summary

Interviews:
1. Medical director of the ED, ED administrator, triage manager

Other activities:
1. General observation of the ED process
2. Extensive review of T-sheets and the facility's leveling process for ED care
3. Concurrent review of ED record documentation and content
4. Shadowing residents during the documentation process
5. Shadowing attending ED physicians during the documentation process

Observations:
1. Facility guidelines require ED physicians to be very specific in documenting a diagnosis for a patient in need of acute care admission. Specificity is lacking in almost one-third of ED patients who require admission. As a result, these patients must remain in the ED until they have a definitive diagnosis, possibly having a less than optimal impact on patient care
2. Patients in need of consult have an average wait time of one hour
3. One interviewee stated that residents are reluctant to write secondary diagnoses on the patient ED record because they do not want to be criticized by the attending physicians if the diagnosis is wrong when patient is admitted to the floor
4. Specific inpatient CDI documentation issues:
    a. Symptoms as principal diagnosis without rule out or differential diagnoses
    b. Medications documented but no documentation of the reason for those medications
    c. Lack of clarity of a diagnosis or reason for patients on ventilators for brief periods

Preliminary recommendations:
1. Conduct ED-specific CDI training for residents, attending physicians, and nurses using ED record examples
2. Design and distribute an ED-specific documentation tool for use by clinicians
3. Consider redesigning templates to include prompters or locations requiring the documentation of diagnoses for medications and rule out or differential diagnoses for symptoms

---

CDI needs to accommodate the patient and the practitioner to create a workable process. Some issues to consider in assessing each outpatient setting include the following:

- Amount of documentation on the record at the time patient is admitted

- Specific times when the physician generally documents in the patient's record during the stay

- How many times the physician documents in the patient's record during the stay

- Availability of the health record during the patient-care process and location of the physician at those times

- Activities directly following patient discharge that may provide an opportunity to query the physician

In an EHR setting, the location of data is less important. However, the availability of the physician is paramount.

Laboratory Outpatient Testing

In the diagnostic laboratory setting, the challenge for the healthcare organization is ensuring accurate documentation by the physician in the order for tests that precede the service being provided. Because effective physician intervention in the laboratory must take place in the physician's office, the healthcare organization must include specific strategies for interacting with physicians and their staff. These interventions may consist of having educational sessions, creating a virtual private network (VPN) or computerized "tunnel" from the physician's office to the hospital registration team, including the physicians in the design of the laboratory order form, and creating specific tools or cue cards to move behavior in the right direction.

Outpatient Testing that Involves a Physician Diagnostician

Outpatient testing involving a physician diagnostician's interpretation of the test results should be differentiated from laboratory testing where results are reported without interpretation by a physician. Examples of these types of tests include radiology, MRI, nuclear medicine, EEGs, and EKGs. In each of these examples, a physician reviews the test results and documents the assessment of the results. There is an opportunity in non-laboratory diagnostic testing to create two interventions. The first intervention is similar to the intervention for laboratory testing where the ordering physician is educated and provided with tools, such as order forms, to ensure the necessary information is documented. The second intervention is with the interpreting physician. Again, the intervention is likely to be with education and documentation tools that the physician can use to document an assessment of the test results.

In some diagnostic test areas, it may be possible for a concurrent reviewer to be available to the physician diagnosticians, particularly if multiple physicians are in one location while reviewing films. The reviewer would be available to answer documentation questions and ask questions (queries) based on information in the reports that are being dictated by the physicians. This scenario may not be possible in many organizations due to location of the physicians and time constraints for review. Productivity for radiologists is intense. The number of tests a radiologist can evaluate is tied directly to the relative value units (RVUs) assigned by CMS to each CPT code for the test. The range of films reviewed per day is estimated to be anywhere from 40 to 175 depending on the level of complexity or RVUs for the test (ARA 2004). CDI program managers should be aware of the structure and process flow of work in the organization's nonlaboratory diagnostic-testing areas. This information can be used to design the optimal CDI intervention for radiology and other diagnostic test documentation.

Physician Office and Clinic Visits

Physician office and clinic visits, with over one billion visits per year, present the greatest opportunity, in terms of volume, to make a documentation impact (NAMCS 2006). A combination of physician education, templates, and other tools should be employed in these settings. Office and clinic visits present an excellent opportunity for physician one-on-one education, if physicians and their patients are willing to participate. This process, often referred to as physician shadowing, involves a CDI specialist with expertise in professional fee documentation and coding. The CDI specialist observes the physician treat the patient. The CDI specialist then documents the encounter concurrently and compares notes with the physician's documentation in the patient record. The CDI specialist and the physician later meet to discuss several patient cases. In the author's experience, the physician practices most conducive to the shadowing process are primary care practices, which may include family practice, internal medicine, or pediatric specialties.

The process works best when the physicians are employed by the healthcare system. Physicians who are not employed by the system, may also be interested in having the CDI specialist perform shadowing and provide feedback about their documentation practices. To avoid any antitrust violations, when the healthcare system provides documentation review services to physicians who are not employees, the healthcare system must charge fair market value for the CDI specialist's services. A primary benefit of physician shadowing in the office setting is that it often engages physicians more strongly in the documentation process than a review of their hospital documentation would. Physicians perceive the shadowing process as more of a personal benefit to them. It is likely that the habits they learn from the shadowing process will be carried over into all of their documentation practices, including the hospital documentation. The physician-shadowing process is both a relationship building activity and a clinical documentation improvement activity. Figure 15.2 presents a list of frequently asked questions about the physician shadowing process. This page can be distributed to physicians via e-mail or hard copy to provide them with a solid understanding of the shadowing process.

Figure 15.3 presents an executive summary of findings from physician shadowing performed for a three-member ED physician group. This reporting format can be used in an office or clinic setting. The summary shows both documentation inconsistencies between what the CDI specialist saw and heard during the patient visit and how the physician documented the visit. The most common finding in the example was that services were performed and diagnoses were discussed but they were not documented by the physician. While shadowing works best in the office and clinic setting, it can also be performed in the hospital.

**Figure 15.2   FAQ fact sheet for shadowing physicians during a CDI assessment and education
session**

Physician Shadowing FAQs

What is the purpose of the program?
Physician shadowing is part of the hospital's initiative to improve clinical documentation to ensure accurate
reimbursement and data quality reporting. The purpose of physician shadowing is to provide feedback to the
physician regarding the quality and completeness of documentation for physician professional fee billing
purposes. Improved documentation in the inpatient record will result in benefits to both the hospital and the
physician. The physician-shadowing process is educational in nature.

How does physician shadowing work?
The physician-shadowing encounter involves a physician documentation and coding expert "shadowing"
or observing the physician during a patient encounter, usually in the office or clinic setting. During the
encounter, the coding expert records all of the physician's activities. At the conclusion of the visit, the coding
expert shares the extent of the physician's activities, how they would appropriately be recorded, and the level
of visit supported by this encounter and subsequent documentation with the physician. There is usually a
comparison between the actual results recorded by the expert and the results recorded by the physician. This
comparison allows for the physician to identify where the documentation practices could be improved to
accurately reflect the care provided.

Who performs the shadowing?
Senior level, credentialed, physician coding experts with the clinical documentation improvement (CDI) team
perform the physician shadowing. These professionals have a significant amount of experience working with
physician documentation, coding, and billing processes.

What is the objective of the program?
To provide instructional feedback to the physician to improve the quality of the physician's documentation in
the patient record as well as to ensure that the physician's documentation accurately reflects the care provided
to the patient.

Service-line-based CDI Implementation

A service-line-based CDI strategy involves documentation initiatives for all patient settings for a particular service line. The primary reason for implementing a service-line
strategy is the belief that it can increase quality of patient care for the organization. There
may also be a focus on increased efficiency. Common examples of service-line management include cancer care, cardiology, neuroscience, pulmonary medicine, and gastroenter-
ology. Management of a service line means that all patient care within these specialties is
consolidated and report to the same manager. Not all care can be compressed into a service
line. Organizations that use the service-line model may have 65 or 70 percent of patient
care managed through a service-line director and the remainder managed by functional
managers like diagnostic radiology and laboratory and pathology services, which treat
patients from all different service lines.

An example of service-line management for cardiology would consolidate the following services: cardiology diagnostic testing, chest pain clinic, cardiac catheterization
laboratory, cardiac outpatient surgery, cardiology inpatient care, and cardiac rehabilitation. These activities are presented to the community as an intense expertise in cardiac
care that the hospital can offer to potential patients. From a clinical documentation perspective, implementation by service line has advantages and disadvantages. The two
primary advantages are increased support from the physicians in the service line and the

Figure 15.3   Sample summary of results for a physician office CDI review

Physician Shadowing Executive Summary	
ED Group: Sample Hospital	
Physicians: Dr. James; Dr. Smith; Dr. Henry	
1. Time period of review	May 1 & 2, 2006
2. Total patients shadowed	21
a. Dr. James	7
b. Dr. Smith	7
c. Dr. Henry	7
3. Records with differences between physician & shadower documentation	16
4. Impact of differences in #3 for facility E/M billing	**+6,083.00**
a. Positive impact	+7,300.00
b. Negative impact	−1,383.00
5. Differences: physician activity not documented	
a. Physician performed a "service" not documented	5
b. Physician identified a diagnosis not documented	3
c. Physician performed a procedure not documented	4
d. Physician provided a drug not documented	2
e. Physician provided a supply not documented	2
f. Other	0
6. Differences: physician documentation not supported	
a. Physician documented a service not performed	1
b. Physician documented a procedure not performed	1
c. Physician documented a drug not provided	0
d. Physician documented a supply not provided	1
e. Other	0
7. Differences: physician E/M documentation	6
a. History	2
b. Physical	3
c. Medical decision-making	1
d. Other	0
8. Impact in #7 of differences for professional fee billing	**267.00**

ability to seamlessly develop CDI in both inpatient and outpatient settings. Physicians are likely to align with the CDI program because, as with everything else in a service-line approach, the clinical focus is the guiding principle. As a result, physicians are more likely to perceive CDI as a patient-care initiative than a financial initiative. Second, the physician and manager support is likely to make transitioning the CDI review process from the inpatient to the outpatient setting smoother as well.

The disadvantages of the service-line management approach for CDI are increased cost and time to implement the program. Specialization, at least initially, increases the number of staff members that need to be trained since they must be trained in both the inpatient and outpatient review processes. In addition, specialization creates challenges for coverage during staff vacancies. Finally, service-line CDI implementation can generally only be implemented one service line at a time to be effective. Therefore, the timeframe for overall implementation may be two to three times as long as CDI implementation that is implemented initially in the inpatient setting and then rolled out to outpatient and other settings. However, service-line implementations may be more likely to stick over time because of physician and clinician support. Since so few programs have been implemented using the service-line approach, it is only possible to hypothesize about outcomes at this point.

Conclusion

Clinical documentation principles are the same regardless of the practitioner or the patient setting. However, for the most effective CDI program, some training components and the review process must be customized for each patient setting. Training should include examples from patient records in each setting with the ability for the physician trainee to identify documentation problems in the examples and make suggestions about how to improve the documentation. The record review process must be specific to both the patient setting and the organization. The outpatient CDI programs most likely to succeed are those that mold the record review process to the existing flow and structure and those that continue to obtain feedback from physicians and clinicians in the setting.

References

Austin Radiological Association (ARA). 2004. Radiologist Productivity and Workflow. http://www.scarnet.net/scar2004/pdfs/SS4_Karnaze_2.pdf.

Centers for Medicare and Medicaid Services (CMS) and the National Center for Health Statistics (NCHS). 2006. ICD-9-CM Official Guidelines for Coding and Reporting. www.cdc.gov/nchs/datawh/ftpserv/ftpicd9/ftpicd9.htm.

Department of Health and Human Services (HHS). 1998. OIG Compliance Program Guidance for Clinical Laboratories. Vol. 63, No. 163. http://www.oig.hhs.gov/authorities/docs/cpglab.pdf.

Department of Health and Human Services (HHS). 1999. OIG Compliance Program Guidance for Hospitals. Vol. 63, No. 35. http://www.oig.hhs.gov/authorities/docs/cpghosp.pdf.

Khoury, A.T., H.L. Chin, and M. A. Krall. 1998. Successful implementation of a comprehensive computer-based patient record system in Kaiser Permanente Northwest: strategy and experience . Effective Clinical Practice. 1:51–60. http://www.acponline.org/clinical_information/journals_publications/ecp/octnov98/patient-record.html.

NAMCS. 2006. National Ambulatory Medical Care Survey: 2006 Summary. National Health Statistics Reports, Nos. 3 and 4. http://www.cdc.gov/nchs/data/nhsr/nhsr003.pdf and http://www.cdc.gov/nchs/data/nhsr/nhsr004.pdf.

NACHRI. 2007. National Association of Children's Hospitals and Related Institutions Emergency Department Documentation Peer Review: Charting Improvements. http://www.childrenshospitals.net/AM/Template.cfm?Section=Homepage&CONTENTID=13034&TEMPLATE=/CM/ContentDisplay.cfm.

NHDDS. 2008. National Hospital Discharge Data Survey—2006. National Health Statistics Reports. No. 5. http://www.cdc.gov/nchs/data/nhsr/nhsr005.pdf.

Opila, D. A. 2002. The impact of feedback to medical housestaff on chart documentation and quality of care in the outpatient setting. *Journal of General Internal Medicine* 12(6):352–356.

Appendix A
Job Description by Example: Clinical Documentation Specialists

by Chris Dimick

With sharp eyes, clinical documentation specialist Sharnetha White calmly combs through a patient's chart. She isn't fazed by the organized chaos that surrounds her in the heart of Mount Sinai Hospital.

White-coated doctors, nurses, and patients pass on the busy Chicago hospital floor as White hunts through charts in search of missing or cloudy physician documentation.

This is White's working environment. The HIM department that serves as her home office just four floors below couldn't be more different. Where the HIM department offers calm cubicles and murmured conversation, the surgical floor boasts unchecked voices, scurrying nurses, and beeping medical equipment. White is in the middle of the action, and that is where she feels at home.

Although sitting down every once in a while would be nice. "One of the challenges is finding a seat," says White, an RN and RHIA. "Down in HIM it is a quiet environment—the patient has already been discharged when the record is down there. On the floor, you have the challenge of the noise, speed, and trying to capture what you want to capture."

White is one of three clinical documentation specialists (CDSs) at Mount Sinai who concurrently review and query physician documentation. Their work is meant to improve clinical documentation in real time, which in turn allows coders to assign more specific DRGs and better portray a hospital's severity and case-mix index.

Mount Sinai implemented its CDS roles and overall clinical documentation improvement initiative in 2004. The change not only improved the HIM department's coding ability and overall hospital revenue stream, it ensured better patient care through better documentation, says Kathy Sauer, MBA, BS, RHIA, director of health information management at Mount Sinai Hospital and Schwab Rehabilitation Hospital.

Article citation: Dimick, Chris. "Clinical Documentation Specialists." *Journal of AHIMA* 78, no. 7 (July 2007): 44–46, 48, 50.

The trend started a decade earlier, and the demand is rising for clinical documentation specialists as more hospitals implement programs, according to Mary Mills, RHIT, CCS, president and CEO of Documentation Solutions in Westland, MI. Both registered nurses and experienced coders fit the role well, making CDS an emerging job for HIM professionals, she says.

Seeking out Better Documentation

A clinical documentation improvement program (CDIP) aims to enhance the documentation presented to HIM for coding and DRG assignment. The program puts CDSs like White on the medical floor to review clinical documents for holes in documentation while patients are still in the hospital. CDSs directly query physicians, asking that documentation clarifications and additions be made in progress notes. In some programs, CDSs even suggest coding specifics, like DRGs, before a patient's chart lands on a coder's desk.

"The physicians are not always in tune with what we need in terms of documentation," White says. "We can only go on the documentation that is provided. We can't assume anything; that is a liability. We can't code off of labs, radiology reports, CT scans—we need the doctor to document."

For this reason, facilities often don't realize full reimbursement for their services. Some coders are wary of an audit by the Office of Inspector General or a denial from an insurance company if they code in full, says Mills. Lacking further documentation, they undercode to remain in a "safe zone."

Hospitals with a high percentage of Medicaid patients rely heavily on proper DRG assignments for reimbursement. Better documentation allows coders to record more specific complications/comorbidities (CCs) and DRGs, which pulls in more due revenue for a hospital, says Mills.

A former coder, Mills has helped design and implement CDIPs at several hospitals since founding her consulting company in 2001. The results of a properly run CDIP are immediate, she says, with improved documentation enhancing both ongoing clinical care and reimbursement.

Better Reflecting Real Case Mix

CDIP implementations have accelerated in the last four years as hospitals prepare for impending changes in the Inpatient Prospective Payment System (IPPS) and the increasing government focus on a hospital's severity rate, according to Laura Pait, RHIA, CCS, senior manager at North Carolina–based consulting firm Dixon Hughes.

IPPS is the DRG system used by Medicare to establish payment rates for hospitalized patients. In April 2006 Medicare announced an IPPS overhaul, giving hospitals three years to transition.

Pait formerly worked with consulting firm HP3 implementing CDIPs at various academic facilities. "You are seeing a new energy and wave of interest" in the programs, she says.

The Medical University of South Carolina has a CDIP story similar to many organizations. After a study revealed that the academic hospital was overly conservative in its coding practices and "leaving money on the table," officials implemented a CDIP in 2004, relates Christine Lewis, MHA, RHIA, CCS, CCS-P.

Better documentation led to more accurate reporting of severity to state officials, which in turn better demonstrated the level of resources required at her hospital. "We are treating sick patients, and our profiling is changing because we are documenting better and making sure we are capturing that," says Lewis, health information services manager in charge of coding and record processing.

Mount Sinai Hospital implemented its program in an effort to better communicate with physicians regarding documentation as well as to "make sure we were attaining the correct DRG assignment," Sauer says. An inner-city hospital, Mount Sinai has a very high percent of Medicaid patients.

One year after implementing the program, Mount Sinai had gained an additional $1.5 million in reimbursement. In the second year, the hospital gained $900,000. "Over time the dollar amount you are recovering gets less and less and less," Sauer says. "But that is a good thing, because you know you are picking up everything you can."

Not only does CDIP improve documentation, it improves the coder's job as well. "This program is putting definite answers to our 'maybes,'" says Andrea Bunker, MS, RHIA, CCS, coding supervisor at Mount Sinai Hospital. "Coders say, 'Maybe this patient has diabetes—their blood sugar shows it, but it is not in the record.' A CDS query can answer that 'maybe.'"

Pait sees the potential for a boost in job satisfaction. In facilities with CDIP, a coder has "improved turnaround time, reduced query rates, and has more complete coding at the time of discharge, which gives a better sense of a job well done."

Coders or Nurses as CDSs?

Registered nurses and HIM professionals are both good candidates for CDS jobs. A mix of clinical and coding knowledge is necessary. In the past, Medical University of South Carolina employed both HIM professionals and RNs in its CDS roles. It now has all nurses, but Lewis acknowledges either profession fits the role. "It is just what you feel is best for your culture," Lewis says. "In our facility we felt nurses may be better speaking with physicians."

The debate is ongoing as to which professional is better suited for the role.

Nurses, who are more familiar with the hospital floor and environment, might be better suited for the CDS role, Pait says. "HIM [professionals] historically don't have that presence in a working nursing station," Pait says. "Not to say we can't be trained and utilized and grow in that, but I think nursing starts off better in that role and relationship when you are staffing your position."

However, experienced coders are more cost-effective and capture more lost dollars than nurses, according to Mills. When working as a coder for a healthcare organization in Dearborn, MI, she conducted a comparison that she says bore this out.

Frustrated that RN CDSs were suggesting incorrect DRGs while on the floor, Mills asked her hospital administration to let her act as a CDS to see who captured more documentation. Mills subsequently helped get information into the record that earned the hospital an additional $245,000 for that one month, she says. In comparison, the RN CDS queried for documentation that led to only an additional $10,000. After six months of similar results, the hospital decided to use coders for the CDS role.

Coders "read a lot of records, we look everything up, we look at the medications," Mills says. The only experience nurses have over coders is working with patients, she notes, but CDSs don't need that piece. "They have the record in front of them that explains everything," Mills says.

Learning Process versus Learning Coding

RNs need to learn CDS processes and coding specifics in order to query for documentation, but coders need only learn the process, Mills says. That cuts the CDS training time in half. "It takes a nurse six months to get on track, just to learn [DRGs and coding guidelines], when a coder who already has that knowledge can just jump right in and start reviewing records," she says. At smaller facilities, CDSs can even code right there on the floor, she notes, shortening the time it takes to produce the bill.

Other facilities look for CDSs who have both nursing and HIM backgrounds. White is an RN and RHIA, and she came into the position with the clinical and HIM knowledge needed for CDS work.

But the job is not for all coders. One must be experienced, have clinical knowledge, and know proper DRG assignments, Mills says. "They have to feel comfortable talking to physicians," she says. "You have to be a people person to do this."

The job is for people who want to get out of the HIM department and interact throughout the hospital, Sauer says. "You get a whole different feeling for how the business of health is done when you are upstairs," she notes.

Exercise also comes with the job. All day, White travels the halls and stairways of Mount Sinai, reviewing patient charts. Sitting down is rare. She usually reads the record standing.

Avoiding a Turf War between CDSs and Coders

Whether a facility uses RNs or HIM professionals as CDSs, it's important to create an environment where CDSs and coding staff can work together. A program cannot succeed without this cooperation, Bunker says.

"If they don't talk to each other, it doesn't work," she says. "They have to work side by side and share their knowledge. There have to be open lines of communication. There can't be turfs."

Territorial CDSs and coders can mean the quick death of a CDIP, according to Bunker. When a coding question arises, some CDSs dig in, saying they know clinical better than coders, while the coders state they know coding better than any CDS.

Mount Sinai took strides from the beginning to combat turf wars, training both the CDSs and the coders on the program at the same time. This demonstrated that their goal was similar, not separate, and that each side should have an open mind, Bunker says.

Coders and CDSs at Mount Sinai also meet regularly to discuss documentation concerns, coding regulations, and other issues. "There is a really good rapport and respect for each other," Sauer says.

Working Fast and on Your Feet

Each morning Mount Sinai's three CDSs mark off which patient charts they will review. Typically they wait until the patient has been in the hospital for 48 hours before reviewing the chart for the first time.

CDSs can't be slow in their reviews. Once they pick up a chart, they are never sure how long they will have possession of it. Although it is important that they see the record, physicians and other providers get first dibs.

"You always have to be looking over your shoulder for someone coming to take your chart," White says. "You learn to share, and it is important to establish a good working relationship with everyone up here. Have an understanding—you have a job to do, they have a job to do."

After CDSs get their hands on a record, their primary duty is to query for additional documentation. If a question is found regarding a physician's documentation, CDSs write a query and place it in the record. The physician is then required to answer the query in the progress notes as soon as possible.

At many facilities CDSs establish a working DRG for each case. CDSs also search the record for any CCs that should be added during coding. "It is like reading a story, and bits and pieces are missing," White notes. "Better documentation allows the telling of the whole story for that patient's length of stay."

While reviewing the chart of a patient admitted for a foot cut on broken glass, White noted that the physician documented that the patient had a history of drug use and was HIV positive. This raised a red flag for the CDS. Physicians tend to use the terms HIV and AIDS interchangeably, but they differ in terms of treatment and reimbursement. AIDS is a different DRG and uses different services at the hospital, and it should be reflected as such in the medical record, White says. Treating the two illnesses can lead to different length of stays and procedures.

Using a customized query sheet, White asked the patient's physician whether the patient was HIV positive or had full-blown AIDS. White planned to check on this query the next day. If the query had not been answered in an update of the progress notes, she would page or track down the physician to get a response.

CDSs also query on the back-end, after the patient has been discharged and the chart has been sent for coding. This is a catch-all for anything missed during the concurrent review, since at times CDSs cannot review a chart due to a short length of stay.

Of course, CDSs can query all they want, Pait notes, but it is up to the physicians to respond if a documentation improvement program is going to work.

Convincing Physicians

Physician cooperation and acceptance is vital to a CDIP's success. "Without it your program will fail," Pait says. "If you do not have an engaged champion selected on the clinical side, you can query till the cows come home and they are not going to answer it."

Convincing physicians comes down to two points. The first: better documentation leads to better patient care. A chart with fine details about a patient's condition and treatment is more useful during subsequent treatment.

"We need a good history and physical on the patient, not just for the capturing of the coding," Lewis states, "but for every healthcare professional looking at the record. They need to have specific and quality documentation for that patient."

Secondly, since better documentation increases a hospital's ability to capture revenue, physicians should be reminded that some of that additional revenue will go toward clinical wish-list items and programs, says Lewis.

Physicians should receive education on the program from the start. It should be clear that CDSs are not querying to influence medical diagnoses or attempting to affect treatment. Their concern is coding, and they ask for clearer documentation to assist in that coding, White says.

A CDIP can take time to grow roots. When Mount Sinai's program was first implemented, physicians answered only 75 percent of CDS queries. Today they answer all of them, Sauer says. Education and acclimation are responsible for the increase. Classes on the program are given each year to the new resident physicians. This helps physicians know up front what to expect out of the program, and that education has helped boost query answer rates.

A physician champion can be invaluable in generating physician support and can serve as an effective liaison between the clinic and coding. Strong support from a hospital's vice president of medical affairs is also necessary.

Bridging the Gap

In addition to coders and clinicians, people with other C titles—CFOs, CEOs, chief medical officers, and chief nurses—must be on board. It must be clear to all of them that clinical document improvement efforts benefit both care and coding, Pait says.

An HIM director must emphasize CDIP is about more than money, agrees Sauer. "Bottom line, it is all for the patient," she says. "If it were my own mother, father, sister, brother, husband, I would certainly want to know that all of their care was completely documented."

Hospitals have always had the challenge of finding ways to improve reimbursement while improving clinical care. Improving clinical documentation seeks to improve both clinical and financial aspects at the same time, Pait says, which is rare for healthcare.

"We thought the clinical and financial were in two different camps, walked and talked to the beat of a different drummer for all these years," Pait says. "Documentation improvement allows us to bridge that gap and be part of the same team, seeking the same quality outcomes together."

Chris Dimick (chris.dimick@ahima.org) is staff writer at the Journal of AHIMA.

Appendix B
The Power of Persuasion: Proven Strategies Inspire Physicians to Improve Documentation

Ruthann Russo, JD, MPH, RHIT

Clinical documentation is the foundation for the codes that link patient care and payment, individual patients and public health data, and much more. The physician is responsible for providing the documentation that the coding professional uses to translate clinical information into these measurable values. And the more complete, accurate, and reliable the physician's documentation, the more complete, accurate, and reliable the coder's final product will be.

Well known resources support the importance of complete and accurate physician documentation, including the *Official Guidelines for Coding and Reporting* and the *Code of Federal Regulations*.[1,2] But what HIM professionals need is a strategy to engage physicians in a collaborative effort to provide this information. In short, physicians have to want to improve documentation. In this article, we'll explore what motivates physicians and how HIM professionals can take advantage of those drives to improve clinical documentation in their organizations.

What Do Physicians Care About?

To formulate a strategy for obtaining physician support for improved documentation practices, every HIM director, coding manager, and coder should first ask, "What do physicians in our organization care about?"

There are certain concepts that are probably important to all physicians, but it's necessary to first determine if certain events in your hospital or community are capturing physicians' attention right now. For example, has a hospital in your region recently been acquired by a for-profit corporation? Has a new group of surgeons been recruited by your administration? These are all things that can affect the way physicians are thinking. Ultimately, the way to achieve complete and accurate documentation is to find the answer to the question, "How can we tie what physicians care about to clinical documentation improvement?"

Source: 2004 IFHRO Congress & AHIMA Convention Proceedings, October 2004

In informal surveys conducted with physicians across the nation, we have been able to put physicians' priorities into the following categories: patients, medical practice, reputation, new technology, and malpractice.

Patients

Physicians dedicate themselves to the practice of medicine because they want to help sick people become healthy and help healthy people remain healthy. If HIM professionals can illustrate for physicians how their documentation practices affect their patients, this will have a positive effect.

In a documentation improvement educational session with a group of oncologists at a community hospital, I reviewed the common DRGs into which their patients were assigned and how these cases were weighted and reimbursed under the DRG system. One of the oncologists became angry that his patients, whom he believed were the sickest in the hospital, appeared to be grouped into fairly low-weighted DRGs. A discussion followed in which the physicians were truly engaged in learning about what documentation they could provide that would make a difference in how their patients records were coded. Focusing on the patients and how the physicians' documentation makes their patients look is a good first step in your strategic plan.

Medical Practice

Most physicians today are still in private practice, meaning that the physician is self-employed or a member of a self-employed group. These physicians may be the most difficult to reach in the quest for improved documentation. However, if you illustrate how good documentation practices in the hospital can affect the physicians' private practices, they will begin to take notice.

Ask your evaluation and management (E/M) coding expert to design a coding session for physicians that will demonstrate how improved diagnostic documentation in the patient's record can affect the level of medical decision making in the E/M code assigned to the patient for professional fee billing.

Reputation

Physicians care about how they are perceived by their peers and the community in which they practice. Community physicians derive their livelihood through patient referrals and other physicians. Given that, tactfully using physician profiling can motivate physicians to improve their practices either individually or as a group or specialty.

In one hospital, the cardiology department was continually profiled as having the greatest opportunity for improved documentation, which meant many cardiologists were poor documenters. The case-mix index analysis was shared monthly with the medical staff. Finally, the chief of cardiology vowed at one meeting that their specialty would be the lowest on the list of "poor documenters" by the end of the quarter. He worked diligently with this department, and month by month, the cardiology group's documentation improved. In this case, the impetus behind better documentation was how these physicians compared to their peers, not whether the hospital was reimbursed more accurately.

New Technology

Most physicians want access to the best technology to treat their patients. If the hospital is willing to share financial information with interested physicians, it can be demonstrated that a healthy bottom line, made possible through more complete documentation, can result in access to better tools for physicians.

This strategy may work only with certain physicians in a community setting who are either interested in financial projections or find financial, analytical information interesting. However, this strategy can be very successful for the hospital that employs physicians. In this sense, the physician's bonus dollars or budget for equipment can be tied to favorable documentation audits or query response rates.

Malpractice

Every physician wants to avoid medical malpractice allegations, especially in parts of the country where malpractice premiums have increased two- or three-fold in the past two years. Here, the HIM professional can link risk management with good documentation practices. It is important to illustrate the connection between complete clinical documentation and patient care quality, which has a direct link to possible malpractice. In addition, the HIM department can also conduct specific seminars on documentation and risk management for the physician. Most medical malpractice insurers have programs that will provide at least a minimal reduction in physicians' medical malpractice premiums if they attend a certain number of educational sessions that address risk management. Inquire with the bigger carriers in your region about whether they would be willing to include your sessions as incentive for the physicians to attend.

Healthcare Data and Ratings

The wealth of healthcare data available to consumers today shines a new spotlight on physician documentation. Patients have several sources from which to gain information about providers, including state hospital associations for state-specific reports, and numerous other Web sites.[3] These data are derived from MEDPAR and other publicly available data sources.[4] The data that are used to determine mortality and complication ratings is your hospital's coded data, which, of course, originates from the physician's documentation. In hospitals that tend to be rated low on the mortality analyses on these sites, it's common that the physicians provide very sparse documentation, especially for secondary diagnoses. Patients with more (valid) secondary diagnoses will have a higher probability of mortality, in general, than patients with one or no secondary diagnosis.

How Can HIM Professionals Make a Difference?

HIM professionals have developed several effective strategies to change physician attitudes toward improving documentation. Try one or more of the following proven strategies to boost awareness of the importance of documentation.

Dinner and a Query

In one organization, the HIM department transformed the retrospective query process into a monthly event that physicians look forward to attending. In this 500-bed hospital, records with incomplete documentation at the time of coding are audited monthly. Retrospective queries are divided up by physician. Then, physicians with one or more queries are invited to a meeting with several of their query peers where, in return for responding to the queries via a late entry progress note, they receive a nice meal in one of the hospital's best rooms. There, physicians are presented with a stack of records that have been carefully combed through by HIM professionals. They can focus on the clinical documentation that led to the query, specifically tabbed and highlighted by the coder in careful preparation for this process. Many physicians look forward to these meetings and have said that they have learned a lot from the process. Interestingly, there are very few repeat attendees, which may mean the query sessions are effective educational tools.

Go Public with Data

By sharing on a regular basis public data about your hospital with physicians, you'll remind them of the important role their documentation plays in such data. If this becomes a regular practice, it can become very positive.

Spotlight a Key Metric

Most hospitals have key metrics that are shared with the hospital management team. Key metrics usually include monthly case-mix index, average length of stay, and census numbers. The case-mix index could be a key metric that is shared with the medical staff to focus on documentation improvement. However, it may actually be more effective to share a metric that is physician documentation-specific. Some key metrics, which other hospitals share, includes concurrent physician query response rate, concurrent documentation audit change rate, and potential for case-mix improvement based on improved documentation. All of these metrics can be shared as one number or by specialty or physician group.

Target Your Education

As noted above, there is great value in providing educational sessions to physicians on documentation improvement and risk management. Your organization should require a minimum number of continuing medical education (CME) credits related to documentation improvement each year. Further, advertisements for documentation improvement CME sessions should clearly state the purpose of such sessions, so physicians are continually reminded about the importance of sound documentation practices.

Make Learning Easy

In addition to offering CME credits on documentation improvement, make the sessions easy for physicians to attend or obtain. For example, offer sessions on cassettes, CDs, or via the Internet.

Talk Doctor to Doctor

To get the greatest success out of any documentation improvement program, recruit a physician employee to assist in the education and query process, because physicians generally relate best to other physicians. The physician liaison can be involved in the retrospective query process, communicating with physicians when there are specific documentation issues that require intervention, conducting educational sessions, and developing and approving coding and query guidelines. Additionally, he or she can serve as a key member of the management team in tracking clinical documentation improvement metrics by physician, physician group, or specialty.

The presence of a physician peer in the documentation improvement process will improve the effectiveness of your program fivefold, and the return on his or her salary will likely be obtained within the first few weeks of his or her appointment.

Know Your Audience

Nagging physicians won't yield the quality of documentation coders need to assign the correct codes. But by examining what motivates physicians, HIM professionals can design documentation improvement strategies that inspire physicians to embrace these efforts.

For More Information

Looking for more information about documentation improvement? Turn to the FORE Library: HIM Body of Knowledge, where you'll find the following articles:

- Authentication of Health Record Entries
- Correcting and Amending Entries in a Computerized Patient Record
- Documentation Requirements for the Acute Care Inpatient Record
- Ensuring Legibility of Patient Records
- How Poor Documentation Does Damage in the Courtroom
- Maintaining a Legally Sound Health Record
- Recommended Regulations and Standards for Specific Healthcare Setting

Endnotes

1. ICD-9-CM Official Guidelines for Coding and Reporting, 2002. Available at http://www.cdc.gov/nchs/data/icd9/icdguide.pdf.

2. 42 CFR 412.46

3. HealthGrades (www.healthgrades.com), DoctorQuality (www.doctorquality), Solucient (www.solucient.com)

4. MEDPAR is the publicly available patient data set that contains all Medicare inpatient claims data by calendar year.

Ruthann Russo (rarusso@hp3.org) is founder and CEO of HP3 Inc., a healthcare consulting firm in Bethlehem, PA.

Appendix C
Case Study: Sioux Valley Hospital USD Medical Center

The Pursuit of Excellence in Medical Record Reviews

by Mary Nelson, RHIA, and Shari Aman, RN, CPHQ

This project was selected as a 2001 Best Practice Award winner. The Best Practice Awards are generously underwritten by a grant from founding sponsor Healthcare Management Advisors, Inc. (HMA), to the Foundation of Research and Education (FORE). Since 1990, HMA has provided compliance and clinical data quality services to more than 1,600 hospitals and 20,000 physicians, and now also provides online solutions via the Internet.

Is your ongoing medical record review (MRR) process producing meaningful results? Are you able to use the data collected to improve documentation and ultimately, patient care? Are your record reviewers comfortable making decisions and able to meet their deadlines? If not, it may be time to take another look at your facility's MRR process.

At Sioux Valley Hospital USD Medical Center, our ongoing MRR program was piecemeal and clumsy. As the largest medical facility in the region with approximately 476 beds, we had 22,438 inpatient discharges and outpatient activity that resulted in 81,002 actual outpatient medical records in 2001. Our MRR program involved members of the nursing performance improvement (PI) council with additional multidisciplinary members to review 30 to 50 closed records every other month with the Joint Commission surveyor's entire record review tool. This process had several shortcomings, including a lack of ownership and meaning to the results obtained. Results were not valued because participants felt that the sample size was too small. Further, tallying and aggregation of results required much validation and re-review of records by the coordinators of the process.

Article citation: Nelson, Mary, and Shari Aman. "The Pursuit of Excellence in Medical Record Reviews." *Journal of AHIMA* 73, no. 6 (2002): 45–50.

We had resisted establishing a new program because of the significant time required. Moreover, we weren't convinced that the new program would be more valuable. However, we recognized the need to change the process when the same problems were found repeatedly in the records, despite calls for action from all departments. Additional motivation came after our Joint Commission survey in 1999. The surveyor identified three issues we needed to address:

- develop our program to provide more trended information

- give more focus to clinical pertinence

- show more documented performance improvement

We decided to design a new ongoing MRR that would be more meaningful to the reviewer and use a more representative sample of records closer to the point of care. The new program became an organizational priority, but no additional resources were available to make it happen. We had to capitalize on existing structures, functions, and resources.

Defining Our Goals

We began by conducting an in-depth review of the Joint Commission standards, scoring guidelines, and intent statements; Centers for Medicare and Medicaid Services conditions of participation; state regulations; and our facility's policies, rules, and regulations. Then, together with the vice president of clinical services and the HIM director, we established goals and objectives for an ongoing MRR process. The goals included:

- define representative sample size for hospital (5 percent was ideal)

- include inpatient and outpatient records in monthly documentation reviews

- incorporate timeliness of documentation monitoring

- provide trended data for analysis and prioritization of improvement opportunities

- provide analysis of aggregate data using Joint Commission scoring guidelines as benchmark

- meet the Joint Commission requirement for a multidisciplinary approach by requiring those who provide the care to conduct the reviews

- shift the focus of reviews to the point of care: the open record

- use the entire Joint Commission review tool and incorporate hospital-specific items and the 19 required elements

- promote action plans and remonitoring to show achieved and sustained improvement

In addition to complete support from management and administration, it was clear that a full multidisciplinary team would be needed to carry out the new MRR process. Our new team consisted of nursing PI council members, representatives from all ancillary areas, physicians, HIM, and PI staff. Further, it was critical to be able to produce department-specific as well as aggregate results for the process to be meaningful and provide desired outcomes. Timely, regular communication of results would be key to a comprehensive process. Finally, this program had to be efficient and simple to implement.

Steps Toward Implementation

Sample Size

Establishing the monthly review sample size to fit our organization was our first hurdle. We wanted to ensure that we reviewed a large enough sample twice a year to start some meaningful trend lines, so we chose to review 5 percent of records monthly, with each team member reviewing 10 records per month for a particular element of the record. Because using additional staff to conduct the reviews was not an option, we had to use existing staff in a more creative manner. We were given the autonomy to design a program that would fit into our existing clinical environment and established workflow.

Timeline

The initial timeline for the pilot study was July 2000 through December 2000. We would then test the data, evaluate the program, and survey reviewers for improvement suggestions. January 2001 through June 2001 completed the second cycle of this first-year phase. By July 2001 we considered our program fully implemented with trended data for comparison and reporting mechanisms established.

Review Tools

To review open and closed records, we downloaded the Joint Commission Hospital Surveyor Medical Record Review Tool. The tool is designed to allow the reviewer to check for the presence or absence of key elements in the medical record. To work effectively with a multidisciplinary group, we needed to reengineer the tool to be more user friendly. We divided it into four sections and assigned each section to two months:

- assessment of patients (January and July)

- documentation of care (February and August)

- education (March and September)

- operative and invasive procedures (April and October)

We knew that verbal orders (May and November) and nursing assessment documentation (June and December) were two important areas for our organization so we developed a separate review tool for each. For the clinical **pertinence reviews**, we developed our own tools to cover the remaining elements on the 19 required elements. Legibility and HIM indicators (documentation timeliness) reviews are addressed outside this structure and the results are then incorporated into the program.

Then, after a detailed analysis of the earlier MRR process, we created binders for the open record review for each reviewer. Each binder included the assigned tool for each month, guidelines for each of the review elements, action plan forms to record any items found that required improvement, and pre-addressed envelopes to submit the original review tools. We initially prepared these binders for a six-month trial knowing that the Joint Commission Web tool changes frequently and to determine which information would be important and valuable to our organization. The binder enabled the reviewers to review their 10 charts anytime during the month, instead of at one designated time.

The focus studies on clinical pertinence involved the members of our multidisciplinary team that didn't have specific outpatient visits, such as the pharmacy, HIM, and PI. This focus group reviews different report types for content on a regular basis and much of the review is done on closed records (the autopsy and donation sections on the required 19 elements by nature can't be reviewed on an open record). The MRR program captures the record as soon as possible after discharge to get as close to the open record as possible. This focus group has evolved as HIM students on their clinical rotations participate in this process.

Next, we established tools to monitor the MRR process. To increase the likelihood of getting solid, factual results, the reviewers needed education and guidelines to follow at every step, especially because there is turnover in PI positions every year. We met with each reviewer, established monthly information sessions, and e-mail and phone "hot lines" for questions and changes.

Tallying the Results

The review tools incorporated a tallying component, which was a manual process throughout the development of the program. Now, we use a computerized tally component for easier data compilation. We learned an important lesson while developing this portion of the tool. Although we give the reviewers only three options for an answer ("N" means that the element did not apply to the record, "P" means that the element is present, and "A" means that the element is absent) and guidelines to make judgments, we initially received many written comments on the data collection tools. This made the tally process more time consuming and we realized the reviewers needed to feel more empowered to make decisions.

At the monthly nursing PI council meetings, we reviewed the results and explored details of the reviewers' concerns. As the reviewers became more comfortable with the review process, they also became more comfortable making their own judgment calls and discussing them. They realized that this new program was an avenue for learning, not criticism. We no longer felt compelled to re-review records.

Tracking and Trending the Data

To make our statistics measurable and trackable, we decided to convert our data into percentages. Then, once the data was ready to be disseminated, we wanted to benchmark it. We also wanted to show the nursing departments how they were doing with documentation each month by giving them an overall score. We decided to "score" each review and compare it to the Joint Commission scoring guidelines as a benchmark (see "MRR Scoring Formula" below). This method proved quite successful, especially at the administrative level. By trending aggregate data, we were able to see the individual departmental improvement opportunities. Directors were encouraged to keep copies of their own department's review results in order to establish their own thresholds and monitor progress by comparing current results to their previous results and identify and address their own department-specific PI opportunities.

By viewing the aggregate data, reviewers could more easily determine if data collection done on their unit was accurate. Because of the open communication structure we established, reviewers were able to ask questions about whether their interpretation had been accurate.

The staff learned that some of the elements were outside their control, but because they affect everyone across the board, we are still comparing like scores. The reviewers and the directors could then also compare their scores to the scores of the other nursing departments. The next time these elements were reviewed, they could see their overall improvement.

An essential component in gathering and reporting statistics is our master review book that includes all record review activities. It incorporates our policy, review plan, the documentation of the percentage of records reviewed each month against that month's discharges, the listing of the members of the multidisciplinary team, the summary checklist for the 19 required components, the schedule for review including the draft for the year's focus reviews, review results, the reporting and action taken, and a final section for evaluation and success stories.

Maintaining Progress

Once we established the review program, we needed ways to maintain its effectiveness and keep reviewers motivated. When a department shows a gap between its actual performance score and the benchmarks, it is documented on an action plan. The action plan form identifies the problem, to whom the problem was referred, and the action taken. Then, a follow-up is planned before the next scheduled review. Additionally, the process enables the department to devise its own strategy and re-review of missing elements prior to the next hospital-wide review in six months.

Occasionally, reviewers are too busy to complete their reviews and do not send them in. To address this complaint, we send e-mails to the directors of departments listing the non-reporting areas after each tally. The directors' follow-up sends a clear message to reviewers that this program is a priority. Equally effective is posting the results in each committee meeting. When a department fails to submit its results, "No Report" is listed next to its name on the results projected to the entire group. This is necessary to keep our representative sample size for the Joint Commission and to get a good cross section of our overall hospital performance.

Another way ongoing progress is ensured is through support from administration. Each month, we report the MRR findings to nursing senate and patient services directors in addition to our monthly hospital-wide nursing PI council meetings. Upper management leaves no doubt that this is an organizational priority now that we have the tools necessary to determine our PI opportunities. All results from the ongoing MRR process are also reported into the medical record committee. Physicians then review the aggregate results and records are brought in for their detailed review. Action for the physician component of the review lies with this committee and the chief medical officer who sits on this committee.

Impact

Looking back, we feel fortunate that the Joint Commission prompted us to improve our MRR program. The benefits we have realized over the last two years with the new MRR program have gone beyond our expectations. One of the major benefits has been increased efficiency in the review process. Because documentation has improved at the point of care, it requires less monitoring. Now, reviewers spend approximately two hours per month resulting in a total review of 400 to 500 records per month. And because the records are reviewed by those who actually use them, there is a heightened awareness of documentation expectations.

Further, the unit-specific results enable staff to aggregate and track their own progress over time. The immediacy of the results promotes sustained performance improvement for a department and also for the entire organization.

The required action plans have increased the effectiveness of performance improvement measures. The best part of the action plan process is that it is easily incorporated into our existing PI program. Denial of problems has been replaced with the realization that there are opportunities for improvement. While it took some time for the action plans to be accepted at the facility, administrators realized the value of promoting the process. In fact, there were several requests to use the same format for other PI activities. Due to the information gained from these reviews and the resulting increased awareness and education, pain assessment documentation went from 84 percent to 96 percent.

We continue to update and revise the ongoing MRR program. Review tools are updated as the Joint Commission revises its tool. Guidelines are also updated as indicated and at the suggestion of some reviewers. Equally important, the results from this process are evaluated monthly and the process itself is evaluated annually with an informal survey sent to all reviewers, Joint Commission chapter committee chairpersons, directors, and administrators. We want to ensure that we continue to provide valuable data and meaningful information. The individual department binders are considered innovative as a result of analyzing existing processes in such detail prior to implementation of this process. Another innovative component of the ongoing MRR process is the ease in developing focused studies. Clinical pertinence indicators are mostly reviewed within focus studies now.

The most exciting part of this process has been the education all of the stakeholders have received. We've heard several comments like, "I didn't know I was supposed to document that!" Complex performance improvement projects involving multiple stakeholders can only achieve success with small, incremental changes. We believe the continuous monitoring and frequent evaluation of this process has been key to our success.

MRR scoring formula

150 (total number of review elements) – 50 (not applicable elements) = 100 (elements that apply)

100 – 10 (absent elements) = 90 (present elements)

$$\frac{90 \text{ (total present elements)}}{100 \text{ (elements that apply)}} = 90 \text{ percent (score)}$$

References

- Joint Commission on Accreditation of Healthcare Organizations. Comprehensive Accreditation Manual for Hospitals: The Official Handbook. Oakbrook Terrace, IL: Joint Commission, 1999.

- The Joint Commission Web site, available at www.jcaho.org.

- Joint Commission Hospital Survey Medical Record Review Tool, available at www.jcaho.org/trkhco_frm.html.

- Balanced Budget Act of 1997. Sec. 4317. Available at www.hcfa.gov.

Mary Nelson (nelsonm@siouxvalley.org) is the electronic medical record project manager and a supervisor in the HIM department and Shari Aman (amans@siouxvalley.org) is performance improvement coordinator in the quality resource management department at Sioux Valley Hospital USD Medical Center in Sioux Falls, SD. To view additional forms and resources from this best practice article, contact the authors via the e-mail addresses provided.

Appendix D
Case Study: St. Vincent Catholic Medical Center

Clinical Documentation: The Saint Vincent Experience

Ruthann Russo, JD, MPH, RHIT, and Maria Muscarella, RHIA

Hospitals throughout the country are conducting reviews on DRGs, case-mix index (CMI), length of stay, carve-out days, and denials. St. Vincent Catholic Medical Centers in New York City was no exception. Using "home grown" systems, the Case Management department worked collaboratively with the HIM department to measure the quality of clinical documentation and its impact on coding and the CMI. Without formal measurement tools to assist, collating the data was labor intensive. Despite this fact, a trend was identified—The clinical documentation did not always adequately reflect the severity of illness of the patient population and, in turn, did not support the HIM coders in their coding endeavors to achieve and sustain optimum quality and accuracy. Ultimately, an administrative decision was made to implement an independent clinical documentation improvement structure at St. Vincent's Hospital.

A multidisciplinary Clinical Document Improvement Steering committee chaired by the senior vice president of Nursing Administration was developed. It included the medical director; chairperson of the Department of Medicine; vice president of Finance; vice president of case management; director of case management; vice president of HIM; director of HIM; coding manager; Information Technology and HP3 personnel. The purpose of the group was to oversee the implementation, monitor the ongoing process, and address all identified issues.

The steering committee made two immediate decisions:

- Clinical documentation improvement (CDI) specialists would report to the director of Case Management

- Recruitment for the CDI specialists would be done internally

Source: Russo, Ruthann; Muscarella, Maria. "Clinical Documentation: the Saint Vincent Experience." AHIMA's 78th National Convention and Exhibit Proceedings, October 2006.

The rationale for internal recruitment was that staff members were already familiar with the medical staff and clinical documentation, and therefore would be several "steps ahead" of someone hired from the outside. This proved to be a wise decision, as the ideal candidates recruited came from Case Management and from the ICU and had significant experience reviewing clinical documentation in addition to established, positive working relationships with the medical staff.

Role of the Medical Staff

A hospital's medical staff is the key to success of a clinical documentation improvement program. The physician's documentation ultimately will determine the coding; and, in turn, the coding is the data that will generate reimbursement, mortality and severity ratings, quality indicators, and research/planning information. A hospital should take a multi-tiered approach to involving the physician both individually and in groups in the clinical documentation initiative. First, physician champions or leaders should be involved with the initial creation of the hospital's specific CDI program. The physician CDI leaders will be most successful if they are involved managers or practicing members of the medical staff. Because of the differences in approach, it is best to secure the involvement of both a medicine physician and a surgeon. Other criteria that should be used to make the decision regarding who the organization's physician champions will be include likelihood of initial and ongoing support from the physician; and how well respected the physician is by his/her peers.

A documented, structured communication plan should be created to ensure the physicians are informed about the clinical documentation program. The hospital needs to consider both content and methodology of communication in designing the CDI communication plan. For content, the communication plan should focus on why the physicians should be interested in participating in the hospital's CDI program and what value they personally will get from this program. The message may be structured differently for employed or house physicians than it is for voluntary physicians. For example, for employed physicians and house staff, there may be an interest in their own severity level curves for the patients they treat; whereas, voluntary physicians may be more likely to be interested in how improving their documentation will help to improve their own coding and reimbursement for their practices.

In structuring the communication plan, it is important to take both a top-down and bottom-up approach. Top-down approach strategies include starting with an announcement of the CDI program to the Medical Executive Committee. This is usually done through a presentation with handouts or take-aways. Each department head is then asked to communicate the information to their department members. The bottom-up approach is focused on identifying the most effective ways to get information into the hands of members of the medical staff. Depending on the organization, this may be through e-mail, hard copy mail, or announcements posted in the medical staff lounge.

Medical staff training and education in clinical documentation practices is the foundation for a successful and sustainable clinical documentation program. Again, the process must be approached with a multi-tiered strategy. Physicians should be educated in groups by specialty. They should also be educated one-on-one on the nursing units, when possible. Explaining the impact of improved clinical documentation to a physician is much more powerful when their own documentation and patients are used as examples. Physician-specific education can be provided on the units in the hospital, in the clinic, or in their offices. And, of course the most powerful education occurs when the physicians sees a personal benefit in documenting better.

The Role of Concurrent Reviewers

The central catalyst in the clinical documentation program is the clinical documentation specialist, also known as the concurrent CDI reviewer. This individual is responsible for reviewing the inpatient record while the patient is still in-house and identifying opportunities to improve the documentation in the record. When an opportunity is found, the CDI specialist communicates with the physician to obtain necessary documentation in the patient record. Whatever your hospital decides to call these individuals, they are essential to the ongoing CDI process. The successful CDI specialist is likely to be a registered nurse with record review experience. In addition, CDI specialists who are already familiar with the hospital and the medical staff will have a higher degree of initial success than someone hired from outside of the organization.

Because CDI specialists are generally not in high supply, each hospital should plan to provide initial and ongoing training to the individuals hired to be the engine of the CDI program. The initial training must focus on an understanding of clinical documentation guidelines as described in Medicare Conditions of Participation. JCAHO regulations, UHDDS and Coding Clinic guidelines. It is important for the CDI specialists to understand the need to obtain documentation from the physician or other practitioner that is legible, complete, accurate, reliable, precise, and clear. The CDI specialist should tracking and measuring their review process and their physician interaction. This process is often omitted from a new CDI program. Omission of the tracking and measuring process, coupled with reporting of those results, is the greatest reason for lack of sustainability.

Role of the HIM Department

The HIM department is integral to the success of a CDI project. From inception, CDI specialists must collaborate with the coding staff. A regularly scheduled meeting for the CDI specialists and the coding staff should be established. During the early phases of the project, a minimum of twice a month is recommended because there are numerous issues that can be identified and resolved early in the project. Some of the key issues that may arise are as follows:

- Are the communication tools effective?

- Are the coders able to identify all of the records reviewed by the CDI specialists?

- Is the information documented and collected by the CDI specialists useful?

- Is there additional information that the coders need?

- Are there any trends (diagnoses, procedures, physicians)?

- Do the records queried by the CDI specialists contain the documentation required by the coders to code the records accordingly?

These meetings will prove to be invaluable in identifying issues that otherwise go unnoticed.

In addition to the concurrent review conducted by the CDI specialists, it is imperative that the HIM department also establish a retrospective query process. As the success of the concurrent queries ultimately rests with the coders, there must be specific guidelines in place. If a concurrent query remains unanswered by the physician at the time of discharge, the responsibility rests with the coder to conduct the necessary follow-up. Additionally, based upon CDI specialist staffing, if 100 percent concurrent review is not conducted, a formal retrospective query process should also be implemented. This process should be structured (with formal coding guidelines in place), tightly controlled, and measured for its success.

Queries should be precise and based on clinical documentation in the medical record that may be ambiguous, incomplete, or conflicting. As with the concurrent query process, communication tools for the retrospective queries, which are diagnosis/procedure specific, should be developed and used. To ensure consistency, accuracy, and pertinence of the queries conducted by the coders, it is recommended that the coding supervisor review all queries prior to physician contact. The coding supervisor should act as a liaison between the coders, the CDI specialists, and the medical staff.

Ongoing monitoring and tracking of queries with correlation to physicians, DRGs, coders, and quality outcomes should be conducted to measure success as well as identify trends and areas for improvement. Based on these findings, plans of corrective action and of education for both the medical staff and coders should be developed and implemented. The value of this education cannot be emphasized enough.

Role of Support Departments

In addition to the CDI specialists, other ancillary clinical staff can play an important role in the success of CDI. When ancillary staff members are tapped to participate in CDI, it makes the program more of a hospital-wide function than a traditional "silo" function. The value of a hospital-wide function is that everyone understands the process and its importance and there is more likely to be an organizational attitude of joint responsibility. Organizations who embrace joint accountability are generally more productive and successful.

The following ancillary groups can be recruited to participate in the CDI program: case managers, nutritionists, nurse managers, unit secretaries, respiratory therapists, physical and speech therapists, wound care nurses, and other specialists. Each organization should design ancillary support based upon the strengths and resources in the organization and in each group. Generally, the case management group acts as a concurrent safety net for the CDI process. Case managers spend a lot of time interacting with physicians. And, if during their conversations, a physician has a question about a concurrent query, the case manager can provide basic information and direction. The same is true of therapists and specialists who may be trained as part of your clinical documentation program.

The key to cooperation from these groups is to provide communication, education, and feedback. First, communicate to the group or group's manager(s) that they have been tapped to participate in the new CDI initiative, which is designed to improve results throughout the organization. In the communication, be explicit about expectations. For example, you may want to state, "we will provide you with some basic training on CDI (may help with their CEUs) and will ask that you act as a 'resource' to the medical staff when questions arise." Education will vary based on the group trained. For example, the case managers may receive comprehensive training while the unit secretaries may receive general information sessions. Once the ancillary staff has been recruited and trained, it is important for them to receive updates about the progress of the program. If the program is doing well, they will feel part of the success. If the program is lagging, they may offer to contribute more with the physicians.

Maintaining Sustainability

Tracking, measuring, and reporting the impact of the CDI program is essential to ensuring a sustainable program. As noted above, many CDI programs have been shutdown because the organization was unable to determine the value of the activities. Tracking and measuring process, generally driven by a computer program, will provide the ongoing assessment of the value of the questions to and responses from physicians. Objective measures of success that can be tracked with a good CDI tool include CMI, CMI by payer, query rate, and response rate. More importantly, these measures can be tracked by service, physician, time period, or CDI specialist. Generating reports by groups or individuals, if managed correctly, can increase accountability. For example, if the department of cardiology is identified as having only a 55 percent response rate to queries, this may trigger action by the chair and cardiologists to comply with queries moving forward. The reason for increased compliance can be as simple as the cardiologists' awareness that their response rate was much lower than other services in the medical staff.

Appendix E
Case Study: University of Michigan Health System

A Successful Clinical Documentation Improvement Program Using RHITs

Gwen Blackford, RHIA, and Deborah Slater, RHIT

Introduction

The University of Michigan Health System (UMHS) is an award-winning healthcare system made up of University, Children's, and Women's Hospitals; 30 health centers; 120 outpatient clinics; the University of Michigan Medical School; faculty group practices; and the M-Care Health Plan System.

The task of obtaining clinical documentation at the point of care in a large teaching facility is challenging. The HIM department at UMHS is using Registered Health Information Technologists (RHIT) to capture clinical documentation at the point of care to improve facility reimbursement, case mix, clinician communication, and severity and mortality reporting, and decrease reimbursement denials.

The traditional model for a clinical documentation improvement program (CDIP) is to use nursing staff because of their clinical background. At UMHS, we believed that by using key coding staff, such as clinical documentation specialists (CDS), we were able to obtain necessary documentation in addition to meeting all coding guidelines.

Organizational leadership provided the stimulus for a CDIP, with the goals of accurately capturing inpatient reimbursement for services rendered and re-assessing internal coding operations.

Source: Blackford, Gwen; Slater, Deborah. "Strengthening the HIM Profession: Implementing a Successful Clinical Documentation Improvement Program." AHIMA's 78th National Convention and Exhibit Proceedings, October 2006.

Program Implementation

The need for a CDIP was identified based on the following:

- Ineffectual post discharge clinical query process

- Lack of clinician education in real time

- Need to obtain clinical documentation in real time

- Documentation needed to reflect the complexity/severity of patients at UMHS

The deficiencies of the process prior to implementation of the CDIP were the lack of HIM staff visibility on the inpatient units, inadequate and delayed post-discharge clinician query process, querying of attending physicians' instead of documenting clinician, and missing the educationa. opportunities during querying.

A consultant performed an internal coding operation assessment and focused on capturing information to drive appropriate DRG assignments for facility reimbursement.

The consultant and the HIM director worked together on the following. rounding with clinical services to understand their documentation workflow process, developing a framework for the CDIP, which included a re-organization of the coding unit structure to create three clinical service teams (Mott, Maize, and Blue), creating new job descriptions for clinical documentation specialists (CDS) and coding compliance and education coordinators (CCEC), and developing a new salary scale. The coding staff was able to apply for all new positions.

The Clinical Information Decision Support Services (CIDSS) unit identified clinical services for potential documentation opportunities based on DRGs without CCs, such as cardiology, neurosurgery, orthopedics, etc.

We used the P-D-C-A (Plan-Do-Check-Act) quality improvement tool to identify the following:

- Problems

- Root causes

- Improvement goals

- Mission statement

Problems: incomplete and/or contradictory clinical documentation, incomplete documentation for facility reimbursement, severity and complexity of patient mix and incomplete specificity of clinical documentation to support treatment rendered.

Root causes: lack of clinician education regarding non-specific documentation, and the current clinician query process was post discharge and missed opportunities for clinician interaction and education.

Improvement goals: capture clinical documentation at the point of care, improve facility reimbursement and case mix, improve clinician communication, decrease reimbursement denials, and retain UMHS's reputation as a high-ranking hospital.

Mission statement: To improve continuity of high quality patient care; to support appropriate facility reimbursement; to accurately reflect the severity and complexity of the patients treated at UMHS.

Clinical Documentation Improvement Program Process

The HIM manager and the CDS presented CDIP to clinical departments and identified who performed documentation for each service—for example, residents, physician assistants, or nurse practitioners. A clinical notification and education tools were developed for each clinical service. We identified a contact for clinical service resident rotation schedules and set up rounding times.

CDSs use wireless laptops with 3M/HDM and all clinical online information systems on the inpatient units.

A CDS admission work list was created in the 3M/HDM system for each clinical service team. The CDS performs case review 24 to 48 hours after admission to obtain the "working DRG." The CDS will determine cases for clinical intervention, such as documentation stating "troponin leak." The CDS will contact documenting clinician (resident, physician assistant, nurse practitioner, or attending physician) by either e-mail, page, or in person to ask for clarification if a patient has an MI (myocardial infarction) and if so, to please document diagnosis in progress note and/or discharge summary. CDS chapter was created in 3M/HDM to capture working and final DRGs, the question asked, clinician query response, the clinician response (yes/no), and the reimbursement difference between the working and final DRGs. The CDS will continue to review the cases to check for a clinician response, and if no response, she will continue to contact the clinician up to discharge. The CDS will not follow cases after discharge. The CDS reviews all payers. At the time of coding, the coder will review the "communication" chapter in 3M/HDM to look for documentation of clinician response.

The CDSs round with each of their clinical services at least once a week. The rounding process allows for the CDS to interact with the clinicians, gain a basic understanding of the treatment plans, and to make themselves visible to the clinical teams. The CDS for the Cardiology service was asked to participate in creating an online educational CD on clinical documentation, which is used on a monthly basis to orientate all new residents to the service. Also, clinical services have asked their CDSs to assist with the creation of online documentation templates.

The CDS works closely with the manager to prepare "Documentation Tip" pocket cards with commonly missed complications/comorbidities. We have worked with the clinical departments to meet their needs, such as placing the transcription directions on the back of the tip cards and adding core measure information on the cardiology cards.

Outcomes

Presentations were developed to provide feedback on the CDIP for each clinical service, which included the following: outlining high complexity DRGs, presenting opportunities for improved clinician documentation, providing case-specific examples of DRGs with and without CCs, and identifying clinician response rates and potential reimbursement. CDS staff members have been asked to present the CDIP at various department meetings. We have found that clinicians are receptive to the front-end query process. Also, there is high level of support from the clinical division chiefs. We actually received applause from the clinical staff after one of our presentations. We created a Quality Improvement Story Board for Quality Improvement month and received an award.

There is improved communication between the coder and the CDS staff. Documentation is available at the time of coding. We have seen a strong improvement in clinical documentation with the implementation of the CDIP. Our residents will rotate to other services, and they take what they have learned and practice it on other services.

The physician query response rate is 90 percent, and the potential reimbursement identified through the physician query process is approximately $5 million.

Next Steps

Since the CDIP has been a great success, our plan is to create one to two additional CDS positions to cover the remaining clinical services. We will continue to monitor outcomes of the CDIP and make improvements, trend pre- and post-CDIP data, review documentation for All Payer Refined-Diagnosis Related Groups (APR-DRGs), work with clinicians on creating documentation templates, and create methods to improve clinician education, such as newsletters, Web site material, and presentations at resident grand rounds.

In a teaching institution, learning is a never ending process, and our goal is to become a larger part of that process.

Getting Quality Clinical and Coded Data: How UMHS's CDIP Improved Clinical Coded Data and Clinical Staff Relationships

by Gwendolyn Blackford, BS, RHIA, and Rosanne Whitehouse, MPH

Obtaining codeable clinical documentation at the point of care in a large teaching facility can be challenging. However, the HIM department at the University of Michigan Health System (UMHS) in Ann Arbor, MI, took on the task, implementing a clinical documentation improvement program (CDIP). As a result of UMHS's successful CDIP implementation, HIM staff and clinicians are well positioned to effectively code under the new MS-DRG system and capture present on admission reporting indicators.

This article details UMHS's program and how it has improved the organization's coding and reimbursement.

Improving the Bottom Line

UMHS decided to implement the program to improve its bottom line. Organizational leaders wanted to accurately capture inpatient facility reimbursement. The program also provided UMHS the opportunity to re-assess internal coding operations.

UMHS identified four areas for improvement as part of its CDIP implementation:

- Improve the post-discharge query process

- Implement real-time clinician education

- Obtain complete clinical documentation at the point of care

- Ensure documentation reflects the complexity and severity of patients treated

Prior to implementation UMHS experienced many of the same inefficiencies in its coding functions that other hospitals experience. There was a lack of HIM staff visibility on the inpatient units. Oftentimes, the only interaction coding professionals had with physicians was through an inefficient and delayed post-discharge query process.

Article citation: Blackford, Gwendolyn; Whitehouse, Rosanne. "Getting Quality Clinical and Coded Data: How UMHS's CDIP Improved Clinical Coded Data and Clinical Staff Relationships." *Journal of AHIMA* 78, no. 9 (October 2007).

Although documentation is done by attending physicians, fellows, residents, nurse practitioners, and physician assistants, the query process was geared toward attending physicians instead of documenting clinicians. Most important, UMHS felt that it was missing valuable educational opportunities for clinicians.

Program Implementation

With the support and strategic leadership of the chief administrator for HIM, a work group formed to identify a consultancy to develop and implement the program. UMHS used the consultancy to assess its internal coding operations and to identify opportunities for capturing information to drive appropriate DRG assignment for facility reimbursement.

The consultancy and the coding manager worked together to develop a framework for the CDIP. They rounded with clinical services to understand the documentation workflow process. They then reorganized the coding unit structure to create three clinical service teams, created a new job description for clinical documentation specialists (CDSs), and developed a new salary scale.

CDIPs often use nursing staff to capture clinical documentation at the point of care because of their clinical background, but UMHS decided to employ key coding staff (registered health information technicians) in the CDS role. This approach not only allows coders to obtain the documentation needed for coding and reimbursement, it also helps develop positive working relationships with medical staff.

The clinical information decision support services unit assisted the HIM department in identifying clinical services for potential documentation opportunities based on DRGs without complications/comorbidities (CCs).

UMHS used the plan-do-check-act quality improvement process to identify the problems, root causes, and improvement goals. The problems included incomplete or contradictory clinical documentation that did not consistently support facility reimbursement, the severity and complexity of the patient mix, or treatment rendered. The root causes were found to be a lack of clinician education regarding nonspecific documentation and a post-discharge query process that resulted in missed opportunities for clinician interaction and education.

UMHS set the following improvement goals:

- Capture clinical documentation at the point of care
- Improve facility reimbursement and case mix
- Improve clinician communication
- Decrease reimbursement denials
- Retain UMHS's reputation as a high-ranking hospital

The CDIP Process

The coding manager and CDS staff presented the improvement program to clinical departments and identified who performed documentation for each service (for example, residents, physician assistants, or nurse practitioners). They also identified a contact for the clinical service resident rotation schedules and set up rounding times.

The CDSs use wireless laptops to capture clinical data at the point of care, and all online clinical information systems on the inpatient units facilitate baseline and working DRG assignment to determine if there are query opportunities.

A CDS admission work list was created for each clinical service team. The CDS performs a case review 24 to 48 hours after admission to obtain the baseline DRG. The CDS then selects cases for intervention. For example, if the documentation states "troponin leak," the CDS will contact the documenting clinician (resident, physician assistant, nurse practitioner, or attending) by e-mail, page, or face-to-face conversation to ask whether the patient also had a myocardial infarction. If the patient did, the CDS would then request the clinician document the diagnosis in a progress note and the discharge summary.

The CDS will continue to review the case to check for a clinician response. If no response is received, the CDS will continue to contact the clinician up to discharge. When the chart is coded, the coder has access to the CDS's notes in the abstract to alert the coder to look for documentation of a clinician response in the record.

UMHS modified the abstract to capture a baseline DRG and any potential working DRGs, the questions asked, and whether the clinician responded. If the clinician did respond, the CDS notes in the abstract if the requested information was documented in the chart. If the query resulted in a DRG change, the reimbursement difference between the baseline and working DRG is calculated.

The CDS staff rounds with each of their clinical services at least once a week. The rounding process allows the CDS to interact with the clinicians, gain a basic understanding of the treatment plans, and make themselves visible to the clinical teams. The CDSs also have been asked by clinical services to assist with the creation of online documentation templates.

In order to facilitate documentation for clinicians, pocket cards with documentation tips were developed, including commonly missed CCs and other documentation hints specific to the clinician's service. In addition, space on the back of the cards was dedicated for clinician requests, such as directions on how to use the dictation system and core measures information for the cardiology tip cards.

Reaping the Benefits

The CDIP team periodically presents the results of the program to each clinical service. The presentations outline the high-complexity DRGs and identify opportunities for improving clinician documentation. The team also provides case examples of DRGs with and without CCs to show the financial impact of accurate and complete documentation. The clinicians are presented with their query response rates. The CDS staff has also been asked to present the program's results at various department meetings.

UMHS has found that clinicians are very receptive to the front-end query process. There has also been greater collaboration between clinicians and the CDS staff.

Using RHITs in the CDS role has created positive communication between coders and the CDS staff. The coding team has benefited from documentation being available at the time of coding. UMHS has seen great improvement in clinical documentation with the implementation of the CDIP.

The physician query response rate is 82 percent. The CDIP team feels it is truly higher than this, as physicians will add documentation at discharge and the current process reports the rate while patients are still in-house. The post-discharge query process has decreased significantly from 819 queries in 2003 to 380 in 2006. The potential reimbursement identified through the physician query process from the point of the admitting DRG to the working DRG to date is more than $13 million.

Next Steps

Given the success of the program, UMHS plans to create additional CDS positions to cover the remaining clinical services. The organization will continue to monitor CDIP outcomes to make improvements to the program.

UMHS plans to continue to trend pre- and post-CDIP data and review documentation for present on admission indicators and MS-DRGs as part of its improvement goals. The CDIP team also will continue to work with clinicians on improving documentation, creating documentation templates, producing newsletters, and a CDIP Web site, and presenting at resident grand rounds.

Gwendolyn Blackford (gmbford@umich.edu) is the coding manger and Rosanne Whitehouse is the chief administrator of HIM at the University of Michigan Health System in Ann Arbor, MI.

Index